DIAGNOSING MUSCULOSKELETAL PROBLEMS

A Practical Guide

D1736542

DIAGNOSING MUSCULOSKELETAL PROBLEMS

A Practical Guide

FREDERICK G. LIPPERT III, M.D.
Associate Professor
Department of Orthopaedics
University of Washington School of Medicine
Seattle, Washington

CAROL C. TEITZ, M.D.
Assistant Professor
Department of Orthopaedics
Division of Sports Medicine
University of Washington
Seattle, Washington

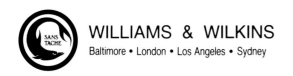

WILLIAMS & WILKINS
Baltimore • London • Los Angeles • Sydney

Editor: Kimberly Kist
Associate Editor: Linda Napora
Copy Editor: Michael Treadway
Design: JoAnne Janowiak
Illustration Planning: Wayne Hubbel
Production: Raymond E. Reter

Printed in the United States of America

Library of Congress Cataloging-in-Publication Data

Lippert, Frederick G., 1934–
    Diagnosing musculoskeletal problems.

    Bibliography: p. 00
    Includes index.
    1. Musculoskeletal system—Diseases—Diagnosis—Case studies. I. Teitz, Carol C. II. Title. [DNLM: 1. Bone Diseases—diagnosis. 2. Muscular Diseases—diagnosis. WE 141 L765d]
    RC925.7.L57 1987   616.7′075   86-11179
    ISBN 0-683-05052-4

Composed at the
Waverly Press, Inc.

87 88 89 90 91
10 9 8 7 6 5 4 3 2 1

This book is dedicated to our mentors who, by example, interest, and encouragement, stimulated us to improve methods for educating students of the musculoskeletal system.

The goal of this book is to help the reader improve his or her skills in diagnosing musculoskeletal problems. Studies have shown that diagnostic difficulties result from failure to obtain adequate data and validate it, from misinterpreting the meaning of data, and from failure to use the data to substantiate or refute diagnostic possibilities. When dealing with musculoskeletal problems, one must also assess the problem's impact on the patient.

This book provides conceptual tools and thinking strategies, along with practical exercises, to help the reader increase his or her depth of analysis of a given problem. The book should be used in conjunction with basic texts and reference sources concerning the musculoskeletal system. Just as learning to read music does not provide one with the ability to play a musical instrument, so learning about the musculoskeletal system from texts does not assure one the ability to solve clinical musculoskeletal problems. Both require practice. The approaches and practice cases in this book will help the reader develop the skills needed to approach a musculoskeletal problem, sift and sort the data, and come to a defensible conclusion.

F.G.L.
C.C.T.

ACKNOWLEDGMENT

Many of the ideas pertaining to problem solving contained herein have emanated from a long association with Dr. James Farmer in his capacity as director of the Basic Course for Orthopaedic Educators under the auspices of the American Academy of Orthopaedic Surgeons.

CONTENTS

CONTENTS

1 Instructions

Instructions

This book is composed of a chapter on problem solving (Chapter 2) followed by a series of cases and flow sheets, which are grouped by presenting complaint (Chapters 3 to 11). The chapter on problem solving provides thinking strategies for eliciting, sorting, clarifying, validating, and processing data. The cases provide practical exercises with the authors' interpretations to compare with your own. The flow sheets provide summaries of the differential diagnoses, natural history, and treatment options of selected disease processes.

Read Chapter 2 on approaches to problem solving. Then select a series of cases with the same presenting complaint and proceed with the first case as follows:

1. Read the case to obtain a general understanding of the problem and the chain of events.
2. Read the questions following the case.
3. Reread the case carefully considering the meaning of each sentence and looking for diagnostic clues and answers to the questions.
4. Consult the flow sheets and other textbooks for more information about possible diagnoses.
5. Formulate a list of differential diagnoses, and try to select a working diagnosis.
6. Compare your interpretation with that of the authors, trying to reconcile any differences.
7. Proceed to the next case in the series and repeat steps 1 through 6.

The cases are real cases from the authors' practices and have been selected as generally representative of a given diagnosis. They are not, however, clear "textbook cases." Some sifting and processing of information is required to arrive at a diagnosis.

The questions provided are similar to questions you might ask yourself when interviewing a patient; they are meant to lead you to elicit further historical data, perform further physical examination, or order additional laboratory tests. The questions will direct your attention to key points, which will help you formulate a list of possible diagnoses. Use the flow sheets to identify key factors that help narrow the range of diagnostic possibilities. Each flow sheet is a skeleton overview of several disease processes with similar presentations. It is not meant to be an exhaustive outline of every diagnostic and treatment possibility but to provide concise summaries of the longitudinal course of several disease processes.

On each flow sheet you will find seven columns. The first of these is labeled "Precipitating Event or Cause." You will notice that the information listed under this column does not "flow" across the sheet as does the remainder of the information. This is true for three reasons: First, each of these items might cause more than one of the problems listed under "Differential Diagnosis." Second, some of these events might be those which bring the patient to the doctor but do not specifically cause the subsequently diagnosed problem. For example, in the consideration of a child with leg pain, one will commonly elicit a history of trauma, as children frequently fall. When the child complains of leg pain, the parents remember that he fell recently and therefore associate the pain with the fall. Don't forget, however, that an infection or tumor might also be present. In other words, although some of the precipitating events or causes should lead you quickly to the diagnosis, others may be coincidental but may have precipitated the patient's seeking medical care. Third, items in this column represent historical factors that you should try to elicit when sorting diagnostic possibilities. In summary, this column contains a spectrum of inciting events or causes of the problems listed under "Differential Diagnosis."

The column labeled "Differential Diagnosis" presents several diagnoses associated with the presenting complaint. It is not meant to include all possibilities but does include common or potentially catastrophic problems presenting with pain of the type under consideration–low back pain, for example.

The "Key Findings" column lists those findings from the history and physical examination that are present in a high percentage of patients with each diagnosis. They do not include all the possible historical or physical findings for a given diagnosis but rather those that help you differentiate one diagnosis from another.

The "Key Tests" clinch the diagnosis in most cases. If the key tests are positive and the key historical and physical findings are present, the diagnosis indicated is highly likely. These keys should open the door to strong consideration of that diagnosis.

Each entry under "Natural History if Untreated" states for the corresponding diagnosis the course of events *likely* to occur without medical intervention.

The information under "Treatment" includes the *majority* of commonly accepted, current treatment modalities for each problem.

Finally "Expected Outcome with Treatment" describes the anticipated results of the intervention indicated. The flow sheets do not include every eventuality under "Natural History if Untreated" or "Expected Outcome with Treatment" but rather are meant to serve as information organizers. You should obtain your information from basic texts and use the flow sheets to help you decide why the patient is likely to have one diagnosis rather than another.

The authors' interpretation of each case is provided in the "Discussion" section following the case presentation and study questions. The answers to the questions are found within the discussion. After selecting a working diagnosis, look up the authors' working diagnosis in the key at the back of the book. Use the discussion to learn how the authors arrived at that diagnosis and to compare your interpretation with that of the authors. You should be able to defend your diagnosis by inclusion or exclusion of pertinent information. "Guessing" the correct diagnosis is not the goal of these exercises. Rather, they are meant to provide practice in gathering, sorting, and interpreting data.

Once you are satisfied with your understanding of the case, proceed to the next case of a patient presenting with the same complaint. Despite the similarity in presenting complaint, careful sifting of the historical and physical findings should lead you to a different diagnosis. Working

Instructions

the series of problems in each chapter, compare and contrast the important features that distinguish one diagnostic picture from another. Studying the cases as recommended will help you perfect your ability to develop a list of differential diagnoses and arrive at a defensible working diagnosis.

2

Introduction to Problem Solving

Introduction to Problem Solving

A patient comes to you with a musculoskeletal problem. Your goal is to solve that patient's problem. As a health professional working with the musculoskeletal system you may assume different roles in this process. You may be the primary physician responsible for collecting and interpreting the data needed for a definitive diagnosis. As a consultant or member of a peer review panel, you may be asked to comment on the validity of a diagnosis or the appropriateness and outcome of treatment. In all these roles, the clinician must have a working knowledge of both the diagnostic process and the treatment process and must therefore be adept at problem solving in the musculoskeletal system. The problem-solving process includes the whole spectrum from diagnosis and treatment to a satisfactory result. The student is primarily concerned with developing diagnostic skills, leaving the details of treatment to be learned in residency. The emphasis of this book is on developing expertise in the diagnostic part of the problem-solving process. This chapter discusses thinking strategies for eliciting, sorting, clarifying, validating, and processing data. In addition the conceptual tools needed for these thinking strategies are provided.

PREREQUISITES

Prerequisites for musculoskeletal problem solving include the following:

1. The ability to perform and interpret a basic history and physical examination of the musculoskeletal system
2. A working knowledge of musculoskeletal pathophysiology
3. The ability to read and interpret routine x-rays
4. A working knowledge of laboratory aids for diagnosis

Working with the musculoskeletal system also requires that one consider not only the problem itself but its effect on the patient's function and quality of life. In no other system does the effect of disease impact so profoundly on the quality of life, which is affected by pain and the inability to carry out important occupational and recreational activities. Chronic musculoskeletal system problems eventually affect the patient's mental status as well as his or her functional capabilities. The extent of the impact depends on the nature of the patient's normal activities. A hip ankylosed at 45° of flexion may be a minor problem for a sedentary clerk but a major problem in a patient required to do heavy construction work from a standing position. An assessment of the problem's impact on the patient's quality of life is made during the initial history and physical examination and requires a working knowledge of occupations, athletics, and a variety of hobbies. Questions relating to the patient's ability to carry out work, social, and recreational activities should be addressed. Observing the patient perform representative activities in these areas will help determine the degree to which the patient has been disabled. The patient's goals and expectations are also an important part of the total picture. The extent to which they are realistic given the presenting problem may determine how well the patient will respond to treatment.

Another important aspect of the problem is the way it is perceived by the patient, the patient's relatives, the insurance companies, and the treating physician. The presenting picture of the patient's illness or disability may be affected by secondary gain factors. For example, the patient may be inordinately disabled considering the objective findings. From such behavior the patient may gain more sympathy from his or her family and more monthly disability payments from the insurance company. The examiner should be alert to this phenomenon. Careful assessment of objective findings and pain behavior will aid in validating the incoming diagnostic data.

VALIDATION OF DATA

During the initial examination of a patient with a musculoskeletal problem, the clinician often considers data provided not only by the patient but also by the patient's relatives and the referring physician. Reconstructing the course of events as accurately as possible is important when assessing whether or not the data obtained fit with the chain of events. For example, an individual being seen for a recent whiplash injury who describes a forcible rear-end collision, yet states that his hat and glasses remained in place during impact, would be subject to some suspicion. The examiner asks the same questions in different ways at different times throughout the examination until the data are stable. Following a rigid history and physical examination protocol can make this task difficult. The ability to perform an examination with flexibility is an important skill that takes practice.

Much can be learned from watching the patient dress and undress, walk in and out of the examination room, and get on and off the examination table. These are periods when the patient is normally off guard and does not expect to be observed. Distracting the patient with questions while he or she is performing these activities is a way of validating data. Complaints of severe hip, knee, or foot pain not accompanied by restricted motion or an antalgic gait are suspect.

As incoming data are processed, the clinician begins to identify diagnostic possibilities. The ease with which presenting problems are defined and solved depends on the order of the problem.

ORDER OF THE PROBLEM

Problems can be classified as either well defined, moderately well defined, or ill defined:

A **well-defined problem** is one for which there is a widely accepted diagnosis and treatment of choice available to the problem solver. Criteria for a well-defined problem are:

A. One solution to the problem must exist;
B. Only one solution is clearly preferable;
C. A small change in the problem results in a small change in the solution.

A **moderately well-defined problem** does not present a single diagnosis and treatment of choice to the problem solver. The problem solver must choose between alternative diagnoses and treatments. Criteria for a moderately well-defined problem are:

A. More than one potentially acceptable solution exists;
B. A small change in the problem results in only a small change in the solution.

Ill-defined problems are those for which there are no widely accepted differential diagnoses or treatments available from which the problem solver can choose. Criteria for an ill-defined problem are:

A. No solution exists;
B. More than one potentially acceptable solution exists;
C. A small change in the problem results in major changes in the solution.

Problems that are well defined for the experienced physician may be ill defined for a less experienced physician or student because they do not have the necessary perspective or information. The diagnostic component of a musculoskeletal problem may range from well defined to ill defined, while the treatment component may vary independently from well defined to ill defined. The physician must recognize that his or her perception of the order of the problem may be different from that of the community because of his or her level of expertise. In the community the standard of care for a given problem will vary as a function of the order of the problem. Well-defined problems generally produce a consensus on diagnosis and treatment. Moderately well-defined and ill-defined problems do not always lend themselves to a standard approach and can be managed in a number of different ways.

THOUGHT PROCESSES USED IN PROBLEM SOLVING

Problem solving requires different levels of intellectual activity. The thought processes involved have been classified by degree of complexity into a hierarchy called the cognitive domain (Table 2.1). Each higher level requires the ability to use the thought processes at all of the lower levels. Cognitive levels 1 and 2 are considered lower-order thinking since they require only remembering and understanding information. Cognitive levels 3 through 6 are considered higher-order thinking because they require much more complex thought processes. At level 3

Table 2.1
Cognitive Hierarchy[a]

Cognitive Level	Intellectual Activity Required
1. Knowledge	Remember facts.
2. Comprehension	Understand the meaning of facts.
3. Application	Use facts to solve the problem.
4. Analysis	Break down information into parts and establish interrelationships for better comprehension of the problem.
5. Synthesis	Devise a new solution for or definition of the problem.
6. Evaluation	Assess the validity of data, definition of the problem, and results of the applied solution.

[a] Adapted from Bloom, 1956.

one must be able to use information to classify and solve problems. At level 4 one gains a deeper understanding of what the facts mean in relation to the problem. At level 5 one thinks innovatively and creates a new idea or treatment. Finally, at level 6, one evaluates the whole process and the end results. This highest level, evaluation, involves mentally stepping back and asking the questions, "What has been happening?" "How are things going?" and "Is the end result internally consistent with the data, with the ways in which it was obtained, and with what is known about the disease and its treatment?"

The following are some examples of clinical activities at each level in the cognitive domain:

Level I: Knowledge: Remembering the diagnostic criteria for and the clinical features of a disease

Level II: Comprehension: Interpreting x-rays, understanding the meaning of joint fluid characteristics, or predicting the diagnosis from the history

Level III: Application: Comparing and contrasting the characteristics of several diseases with the data at hand and arriving at a diagnosis

Level IV: Analysis: Deriving a more comprehensive understanding of the problem by relating each piece of data and what is known from the literature to the proposed diagnosis

Level V: Synthesis: Formulating a new concept about what is happening to the patient, i.e., a new idea about the nature of the problem

Level VI: Evaluation: Deciding whether the final diagnosis is internally consistent with the data obtained and with known pathophysiology

A dynamic model of the cognitive domain as used in the problem-solving process is shown in Figure 2.1.

The clinician working with the musculoskeletal system functions at the application or problem-solving level of the cognitive domain. He or she reaches down into the lower levels of the cognitive domain to understand the problem or gain more knowledge about it, and up into the higher levels to look at the problem in a different way or devise a new way of handling it, and then to check on how things are going. At time T_2 in the figure, a working diagnosis of a fractured radius has been made. Reaching to the lower and upper levels of the cognitive domain results in x-rays being obtained and interpreted. A definitive diagnosis has been reached at time T_3. The same process is used to select and apply treatment and to

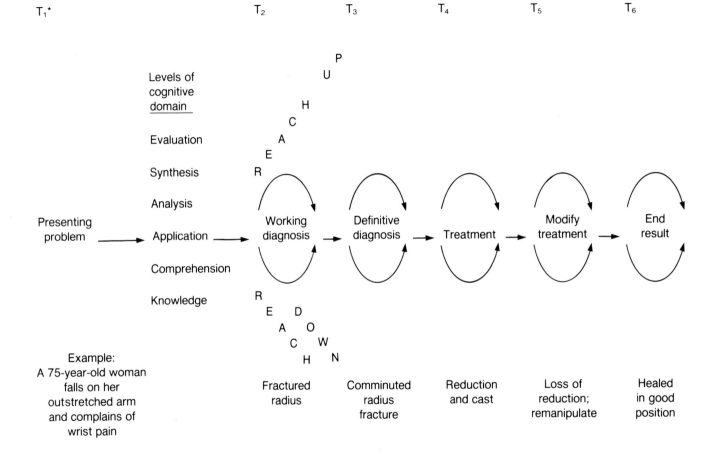

Figure 2.1   Problem solving and the cognitive domain

* Time 1—Initial presentation

evaluate the end result. One uses all levels of the cognitive domain throughout the musculoskeletal problem-solving process.

DIAGNOSTIC APPROACHES

The diagnostic side of musculoskeletal problem solving, emphasized in this book, can be approached in several ways (Table 2.2).

Traditional

The traditional approach to diagnostic problems involves obtaining a history, performing a physical examination, and evaluating x-rays and available laboratory data, in that order. In most schools, medical students learn the pathophysiology of various disease processes and initially have difficulty recognizing the disease from its clinical manifestations, particularly if the patient's disease process is in its early stages and the manifestations are not florid. Many problems present with similar symptoms and signs. Thus, the dilemma medical students often face is that of performing a comprehensive examination while remaining attentive to the diagnostic possibilities causing

Table 2.2
Diagnostic Approaches

1. Traditional
2. Vectoring
3. Pattern recognition
   a. Eliminating the unlikely (rule out)
   b. Including the probable (rule in)

the patient's problem. It is difficult to remember all the right questions to ask in the appropriate order, while at the same time trying to sort historical and physical findings. The beginning student often is so concerned with the sequence and details of the examination format that consideration of the case itself is postponed until all the data are collected. Experienced clinicians know when to abbreviate, modify, or leave out much of the comprehensive examination and focus on the presenting problem. Although the beginning student should learn the standard examination format and sequence so that nothing is overlooked, we believe that vectoring skills should also be learned and practiced.

Vectoring

Following a directional stimulus toward a diagnostic possibility is called vectoring. As the examiner listens to and examines the patient, certain historical data or physical findings may trigger an idea about the patient's problem, which encourages further exploration in a specific direction. This process is similar to a radio compass in an airplane. When the pilot turns on the instrument a pointer immediately swings toward the transmitting radio station. Similar directional signals perceived by the physician should be heeded and used in conducting the examination.

Pattern Recognition

A clinician may immediately recognize a problem from previous experience or because the patient's presentation

Introduction to Problem Solving

of the problem includes so many of the known components of that problem—"a classic textbook case." The physician then reaches up in the cognitive domain to the evaluation level to make certain he or she has correctly identified the pattern. In so doing the physician may use one of two strategies. One strategy is to eliminate diagnostic possibilities that are obviously wrong or are so rare or statistically improbable that they can be eliminated. The other strategy is to focus on those diagnostic possibilities that have a high probability of being correct and to evaluate whether the data collected fit these possibilities.

A helpful method for the student who is trying to learn nontraditional problem-solving approaches is to begin with the traditional approach, but always to keep in mind two likely diagnostic possibilities, attempting to validate (rule in) or invalidate (rule out) these possibilities as the examination progresses. If these diagnoses are ruled out, then two more should be considered, and so forth until the examination is completed. The skillful clinical problem solver must be open minded and sensitive to the unique set of circumstances that surround a particular patient. Obviously some flexibility in thinking and in the examination format is desirable. Using any approach, by the end of the examination one should have formulated a differential diagnosis that is supported by the data base. The next task is to arrive at a working diagnosis.

ARRIVING AT A WORKING DIAGNOSIS

Arriving at a working diagnosis involves all of the prerequisites, thinking strategies, and problem-solving approaches already mentioned. The physician must compare each diagnostic possibility with all of the data and with what is known about the disease entities. Pattern recognition and vectoring are two common examples of the thinking processes used. The working diagnosis really is a hypothesis, which requires further testing and observations to be confirmed or refuted. When the problem is ill defined a more comprehensive and sequential evaluation of the data (the traditional approach) is recommended. Well-defined problems can often be approached more directly (pattern recognition). For moderately difficult problems one might begin with a comprehensive workup but be ready to vector toward promising diagnostic possibilities. The working diagnosis and treatment plan must be based on validated data and take into account the impact of the musculoskeletal problem on the patient's quality of life.

SUMMARY

A variety of prerequisites, thinking strategies, and interview examination techniques have been presented to help the reader diagnose musculoskeletal problems. Although each level of the cognitive domain has been defined and presented as a separate or isolated thought process, in practice the physician has to use all levels concurrently in order to progress through the problem in a responsible manner. We recommend developing an examination style that is adaptable to the circumstances. The examiner should be flexible enough to follow promising leads when they occur. These techniques will enhance the examiner's efficiency and ensure that a valid data base is obtained. The differential diagnosis may be developed from the data base concurrently with the examination. The examiner selects from these diagnostic possibilities a working diagnosis, which may subsequently be changed or modified upon further analysis of the problem and the results of tests and observation. Being adept at musculoskeletal problem solving requires skillful functioning at all levels of the cognitive domain and the ability to use many problem-solving approaches. Developing these skills and techniques takes practice. Working through the case histories presented in this book will provide the student with an opportunity to develop and refine his or her problem-solving skills. These skills provide the foundation for optimal performance in musculoskeletal problem solving.

SUGGESTED READINGS

Bloom, B.S. *Taxonomy of Educational Objectives, Classification of Educational Goals. Handbook I: Cognitive Domain.* David McKay, New York, 1956.
Bucholz, R., Lippert, F.G., Wenger, D., and Ezaki, M. *Orthopaedic Decision Making.* B.C. Decker, Philadelphia; C.V. Mosby, St. Louis, 1984.
Cutler, P. *Problem Solving in Clinical Medicine: From Data to Diagnosis.* Williams & Wilkins, Baltimore, 1979.
Lippert, F.G., and Farmer, J. *Psychomotor Skills in Orthopaedic Surgery.* Williams & Wilkins, Baltimore, 1984.

CLINICAL PROBLEM-

SOLVING EXERCISES

3   Hip Pain

Hip Pain (Adult)

Precipitating Event or Cause	Differential Diagnosis	Key Findings	Key Tests	Natural History if Untreated	Treatment	Expected Outcome with Treatment
Trauma Fall Previous fracture or dislocation Increased activity Lifting heavy weight Chronic alcoholism Endogenous source of infection (e.g., urinary tract, teeth) Insidious (no overt event)	DJD	Activity-related pain	X-ray	Progressive impairment	NSAID Cane	Slowly progressive impairment
					THR	Initial pain relief Loosening after 12 years
	AVN	History of steroid use, excessive alcohol use, exposure to abnormal atmospheric pressures	Bone scan CT MRI	Progressive impairment	Transtrochanteric osteotomy Graft Core decompression	Salvage if prior to deformation
					Endoprosthesis	Pain at 5–7 years
					THR	Initial pain relief Loosening at 10–12 years
	Gout	Positive history (increased with stress)	Crystals in joint fluid Increased serum uric acid	Intermittent flares Joint destruction Tophi	Acute: Colchicine NSAID Chronic: Uricosuric Allopurinol	Intermittent flares
					THR	Initial pain relief Loosening at 10–12 years
	RA	Morning stiffness Polyarticular involvement	Positive RF ANA	Progressive (70%) Intermittent or resolution (30%)	NSAID Steroids Penicillamine	Progression or pain relief
					THR	Pain relief possible contracture

DJD, degenerative joint disease; NSAID, nonsteroidal anti-inflammatory drugs; THR, total hip replacement; CT, computed tomography; MRI, magnetic resonance imaging; AVN, avascular necrosis; RF, rheumatoid factor; RA, rheumatoid arthritis; ANA, antinuclear antibodies.

Hip Pain (Adult)

Precipitating Event or Cause	Differential Diagnosis	Key Findings	Key Tests	Natural History if Untreated	Treatment	Expected Outcome with Treatment

Trauma
  Fall
  Previous fracture or dislocation
Increased activity
Lifting heavy weight
Chronic alcoholism
Endogenous source of infection (e.g., urinary tract, teeth)
Insidious (no overt event)
	Spondyloarthropathies (e.g., ankylosing spondylitis, psoriasis, enteropathies)	Decreased chest expansion	Positive HLA-B-27 Bamboo spine (late)	Progressive ankylosis	THR	Risk of heterotopic ossification with decreased range of motion

	Infection	Very painful range of motion	Joint fluid culture	Progressive destruction	Drainage Resection of infected tissue	Varying reduction in range of motion
	Synovial osteochondromatosis	Catching	Synovial biopsy Arthrogram	Progressive cystic destruction	Synovectomy	Recurrence
	(Stress) fracture	Recent increased activity Impact pain	Scan (x-ray)	Healing Possible displacement	Crutches Pins/nail	Healing
	L3–4 root impingement	Decreased knee jerk Weak quadriceps Positive reverse SLR sign	EMG Myelogram	Gradual resolution or progressive deficit	Bed rest Laminectomy	Intermittent back pain or resolution
	Trochanteric bursitis	Tender trochanter Painful active abduction or passive adduction	None	Resolution	NSAID Injection	Resolution
	Femoral neck fracture	Impact pain	X-ray	Displacement	Nailing	Healing Possible AVN
					Endoprosthesis	Pain at 5–7 years
	Iliopsoas tendinitis	Increased activity Pain on internal rotation against resistance	None	Resolution	NSAID Rest	Resolution

THR, total hip replacement; EMG, electromyography; SLR, straight leg raising; NSAID, nonsteroidal anti-inflammatory drugs; AVN, avascular necrosis.

HISTORY

A.B. is a 55-year-old white male who has worked as a concrete layer for the past 20 years. He complains of "pain in both hips" over a 5-year period. There is no history of trauma or childhood hip problems. The right hip has become increasingly painful and is limiting his work as a heavy laborer. The pain is present at rest, becomes more noticeable toward the end of the day, and increases steadily through the course of a work week. It never awakens him at night. He feels pain predominantly in the right groin and occasionally in the buttock and the medial part of the right knee.

The patient can sit for only 15 minutes before he becomes uncomfortable. He is able to walk up and down stairs but has groin pain when doing so. He has great difficulty reaching his shoes and socks. In the past, aspirin and indomethacin (Indocin) have provided some pain relief. For appearance's sake he has refused crutches or a cane.

PHYSICAL EXAMINATION

The patient walks with a mild abductor lurch to the right and with no apparent discomfort. He stands erect and has equal leg lengths. He has a positive Trendelenburg's sign on the right. He has full painless range of motion of his back and no tenderness to percussion of his spine. He is able to walk on his toes and heels.

Neurological examination of the seated patient reveals no sensory or motor deficits, normal deep tendon reflexes at both knees, and slightly decreased deep tendon reflexes at both ankles. The posterior tibial pulses are 2+ bilaterally; the dorsalis pedis pulse is not palpable on the left.

With the patient supine, the Thomas test reveals a 10° flexion contracture on the right and further flexion to 100°. Flexion of the left hip is from 0° to 120°. The patient has 15° abduction of the right leg and 20° of the left. He has 5° adduction of the right leg and 25° of the left. Attempted rotation of the right hip produces pain and only a toggle of motion, whereas the left hip has a 20° painless arc of rotation. Straight leg raising tests are negative bilaterally.

LABORATORY FINDINGS

Laboratory data include a hematocrit of 45, white blood cell count of 6,300, uric acid 4.9, calcium 9.5, and phosphorus 4.0. An AP x-ray of the pelvis was obtained (Fig. 3.1).

QUESTIONS

1. How do you distinguish systemic inflammatory disease from a localized process?
2. What factors should be considered when evaluating the complaint of pain in this patient?
   A. How do you assess the severity of pain in this patient?
   B. What functional limitation(s) does the problem present to the patient?
   C. Is the problem related to the patient's occupation?

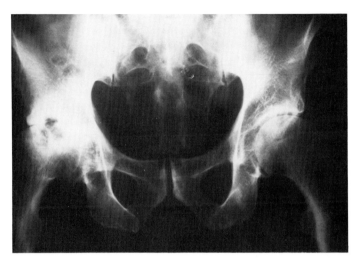

Figure 3.1

D. How do you differentiate pain originating in the hip from pain originating in the spine?
3. How are the following used in the assessment of the patient with "hip" pain?
A. Trendelenburg's sign
B. Abductor lurch
C. Thomas test
4. Given this laboratory work and the x-ray findings, which diagnoses can you exclude?
5. What other laboratory work would help narrow your differential diagnosis?

Discussion

HISTORY

A.B. is a 55-year-old white male who has worked as a concrete layer for the past 20 years. He complains of "pain in both hips" over a 5-year-period. The patient's occupation is physically demanding and requires frequent stooping and heavy lifting. This might produce progressive wear and tear in the back and lower extremity joints. **There is no history of trauma or childhood hip problems.** His problem is not a residual of previous fracture or hip dislocation. There is no history of congenitally dislocated hip, Legg-Calvé-Perthes disease, or slipped capital femoral epiphysis, common childhood hip problems producing structural abnormalities in adulthood. **The right hip has become increasingly painful and is limiting his work as a heavy laborer.** This suggests a progressive condition that is significant in that it has limited his ability to work. **The pain is present at rest, becomes more noticeable toward the end of the day, and increases steadily through the course of a work week. It never awakens him at night.** The rest pain is a measure of the severity of the pain; however, it is not so severe that it awakens him at night. The exacerbation of his pain with activity is a characteristic found often in degenerative joint disease. **He feels pain predominantly in the right groin and occasionally in the buttock and the medial part of the right knee.** This pain pattern is typical of hip disease. Hip disease is most often felt in the groin, with

21

occasional radiation to the medial part of the knee due to the course of the obturator nerve. It can also present in the gluteal and trochanteric areas. Pain originating in the back can present in the same locations but typically presents in the buttock. Moreover, patients who say they have "hip" pain usually point to the buttocks and often have a problem originating in the back. **The patient can sit for only 15 minutes before he becomes uncomfortable. He is able to walk up and down stairs but has groin pain when doing so.** Again these are both measures of pain severity and cross-validate the above information on the severity and location of the problem. **He has great difficulty reaching his shoes and socks.** This suggests a limited range of motion in the hip. **In the past aspirin and indomethacin (Indocin) have provided some pain relief. For appearance's sake he has refused crutches or a cane.** This is a measure of the severity of the problem. Anti-inflammatory drugs have not provided complete relief, yet the pain has not been severe enough to require narcotics. The patient's functional limitations include his inability to work, rest comfortably, or dress easily.

PHYSICAL EXAMINATION

The patient walks with a mild abductor lurch to the right and with no apparent discomfort. Hip pain is related to forces on the femoral head. Lurching to the right shifts the center of gravity over the right hip, thereby lessening the abductor muscle forces. Patients often unconsciously adopt this gait pattern because it reduces hip pain. Lurching can also be secondary to abductor weak-

ness on the ipsilateral side. **He stands erect and has equal leg lengths.** These findings rule out significant joint contractures, spinal deformity, and marked structural changes of the hip. All of these can produce true or apparent leg length discrepancies. **He has a positive Trendelenburg's sign on the right.** Trendelenburg's sign reflects weak hip abductors. **He has full painless range of motion of his back and no tenderness to percussion of his spine. He is able to walk on his toes and heels. Neurological examination of the seated patient reveals no sensory or motor deficits, normal deep tendon reflexes at both knees, and slightly decreased deep tendon reflexes at both ankles. The posterior tibial pulses are 2+ bilaterally; the dorsalis pedis pulse is not palpable on the left.** These findings essentially eliminate the patient's back as a source of his pain. The decreased deep tendon reflexes at both ankles are not an uncommon finding in older patients. Furthermore, the symmetrical decrease makes a neurologic origin unlikely. **With the patient supine, the Thomas test reveals a 10° flexion contracture on the right and further flexion to 100°.** In the presence of a hip flexion contracture, the involved hip will flex as the lumbar spine is flattened, (See Glossary for description of Thomas test.) **Flexion of the left hip is from 0° to 120°. The patient has 15° abduction of the right leg and 20° of the left. He has 5° adduction of the right leg and 25° of the left. Attempted rotation of the right hip produces pain and only a toggle of motion, whereas the left hip has a 20° painless arc of motion.** These findings localize the problem to the hip. **Straight**

leg raising tests are negative bilaterally. Pain originating from the back is less likely.

LABORATORY FINDINGS

Laboratory data include a hematocrit of 45, white blood cell count of 6,300, uric acid 4.9, calcium 9.5, and phosphorus 4.0. An AP x-ray of the pelvis was obtained (Fig 3.1). These normal laboratory data in addition to the x-ray findings of joint space narrowing, sclerosis, and cyst formation exclude the inflammatory arthritides, infection, and avascular necrosis. A normal erythrocyte sedimentation rate (ESR) would eliminate the diagnosis of an active inflammatory process. Back films would allow identification of structural abnormalities that may produce pain. A normal uric acid does not exclude gout.

HISTORY

The patient is a 40-year-old white male truck driver complaining of left groin pain and hip stiffness of 1 year's duration. After a long drive his hip becomes stiff, creating difficulties getting in and out of the cab of his truck. Three years ago he sustained a head injury and fractured wrist in a motor vehicle accident. He was comatose and required corticosteroids for approximately 1 week. After recovering from this accident he did well until 1 year ago when he began to experience left groin pain. The discomfort level has remained constant, but the stiffness has since increased markedly. The pain is aggravated by walking, driving, and sitting for long periods of time. He is otherwise in good health.

PHYSICAL EXAMINATION

Physical examination reveals an antalgic gait favoring the left leg, as well as a short leg gait on the left. When standing on the involved leg the patient has a negative Trendelenburg's sign. Palpation of the iliac crests when the patient is standing reveals that the left is ½ inch lower than the right. When the patient is supine, leg length measurements and hip range of motion are as follows:

Leg length measurement (inches):	Left	Right
Anterior superior iliac spine to medial malleolus	35	35
Umbilicus to medial malleolus	40	39

Hip range of motion:	Left	Right
Flexion	30–90°	0–125°
Abduction	30°	35°
Adduction	0	20°
External rotation (supine, knee extended)	20°	30°
Internal rotation (supine, knee extended)	10°	15°

Lumbar spine and lower extremity neurologic examination are normal.

LABORATORY FINDINGS

An AP x-ray of the patient's pelvis was taken (Fig 3.2).

QUESTIONS

1. How do you account for the time interval between the accident and the current symptoms?
2. Given the antalgic gait, why is the Trendelenburg's sign negative?
3. What factors affect apparent leg length? How do the findings explain this patient's short leg gait?
4. While walking, how does this patient compensate for his hip flexion contracture?
5. What further workup would be helpful in distinguishing the possible diagnoses?

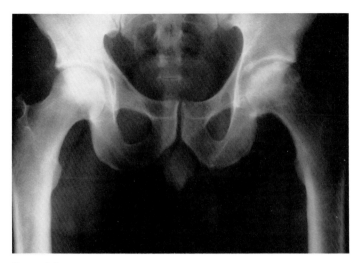

Figure 3.2

Discussion

HISTORY

The patient is a 40-year-old white male truck driver complaining of left groin pain and hip stiffness of 1 year's duration. Hip problems often present with groin pain. **After a long drive his hip becomes stiff, creating difficulties getting in and out of the cab of his truck.** The increasing stiffness after relative immobilization sug-gests an arthritic process. **Three years ago he sustained a head injury and fractured wrist in a motor vehicle accident. He was comatose and required corticosteroids for approximately 1 week.** He may have sustained a hip injury in the same accident. High-dose steroids are associated with avascular necrosis of the femoral head. **After recovering from this accident he did well until 1 year ago when he began to experience left groin pain.** The time interval between the accident and the pain suggests that a traumatic hip injury did not occur at the time of the accident. Avascular necrosis of the femoral head could have begun at that time but not become sympto-matic until 1 year later. Although avascular necrosis sometimes becomes painful shortly after it occurs, in other cases pain does not begin until the avascular seg-ment has collapsed, causing incongruity in the joint. **The discomfort level has remained constant, but the stiffness has since increased markedly.** This suggests the onset of secondary arthritis. **The pain is aggravated by walking, driving, and sitting for long periods of time.** Activity-related pain as well as pain after relative immobilization are consistent with an arthritic process.

PHYSICAL EXAMINATION

Physical examination reveals an antalgic gait favoring the left leg, as well as a short leg gait on the left. The patient is splinting the involved side. The short leg gait may be due to a true short left leg or to a left hip or knee contracture. **When standing on the involved leg the pa-tient has a negative Trendelenburg's sign.** It is unusual

25

for a patient with hip pain to have a negative Trendelenburg's sign. **Palpation of the iliac crests when the patient is standing reveals that the left is ½ inch lower than the right.** The left leg may be shorter than the right, or there may be a left hip or knee contracture. **When the patient is supine, leg length measurements and hip range of motion are as follows: (See leg length measurements.)** The distance from the anterior superior iliac spine to the medial malleolus is a measure of the true leg length. In this case the true leg lengths are equal (35 inches). The distance from the umbilicus to the medial malleolus measures apparent leg length. In this case the left leg is apparently longer than the right. Although the findings on supine and standing examination appear to be inconsistent, apparent leg length can be affected by actual leg length, contractures, and pelvic obliquity. An additional estimate of apparent leg length to determine whether shortening is in the thigh or the leg can be obtained by flexing the hips and knees to 90° and comparing the heights of the knees from the examination table. If the femur is shorter on one side than the other, the knees will be at different levels. **(See hip range of motion.)** In general, flexion or adduction contractures will produce apparent shortening. Abduction contractures will produce apparent lengthening. In this case, the 30° flexion

contracture explains the findings in gait and stance, during which the left leg appears shorter despite the fact that the leg lengths are equal. The left abduction contracture (failure to adduct) explains the apparent increase in left leg length when measured in the supine position. It also explains the negative Trendelenburg's sign. One must be able to adduct the involved hip to have a Trendelenburg's sign. The decrease in rotation is a sign of early degenerative joint disease. **Lumbar spine and lower extremity neurologic examination are normal.** Pain originating from lumbar nerve roots can simulate hip pain. However, the signs on physical examination will be different. Generally, no signs of hip disease such as limited range of motion will be present.

LABORATORY FINDINGS

An AP x-ray of the patient's pelvis was taken (Fig 3.2). The pelvic x-ray reveals a "crescent sign," indicating separation of the subchondral bone of the left femoral head, consistent with avascular necrosis.

Bone scan, CT, and MRI are often useful in differentiating avascular necrosis from inflammatory or infectious processes.

HISTORY

A.G. is a 78-year-old sedentary woman who presents with right groin pain, which has been present for 3 days. Three days ago in her home she slipped on a throw rug but managed to catch herself and did not fall to the floor. Since that time, however, she has noted some groin pain and has been limping slightly. In addition, pain has created difficulty getting in and out of bed as well as in and out of the bathtub. She has a history of a vertebral compression fracture 3 years ago after a fall in the bathroom.

PHYSICAL EXAMINATION

Physical examination reveals a frail elderly woman who is limping with a lurch over the right hip. She has a positive Trendelenburg's sign on the right (Fig 3.3). The range of motion of her hips is essentially symmetrical. However, the patient guards and has slight pain with internal rotation of her right hip. Percussion of either the right greater trochanter or the heel produces pain in the right groin. The patient cannot lift her right leg off the bed when her knee is extended. Alignment of both lower extremities appears normal.

LABORATORY FINDINGS

An AP x-ray of the affected hip is shown in Fig 3.4.

QUESTIONS

1. What factors might contribute to this woman's frequent falls?

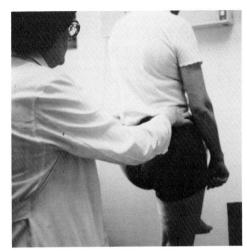

Figure 3.3

2. Of what significance is the past history of vertebral compression fracture?
3. Of what significance are a gluteus medius lurch, a positive Trendelenburg's sign, and inability to "straight leg raise"?
4. What are the pathomechanics of this fracture? How could the fracture have occurred without a direct blow to the hip?
5. What precautions would you advise while the patient awaits definitive treatment?

27

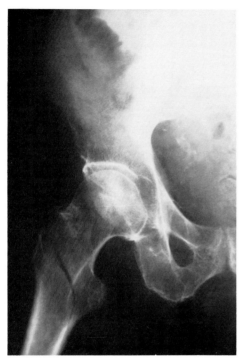

Figure 3.4

Discussion

HISTORY

A.G. is a 78-year-old sedentary woman who presents with right groin pain, which has been present for 3 days. Hip disease is most often felt in the groin. **Three days ago in her home she slipped on a throw rug but managed to catch herself and did not fall to the floor. Since that time, however, she has noted some groin pain and has been limping slightly.** This is a typical history for femoral neck fracture in the elderly. The uncoordinated muscle contractions sustained trying to regain balance produce sufficiently strong forces to fracture an osteopenic femoral neck. **In addition, pain has created difficulty in getting in and out of bed as well as in and out of the bathtub.** The pain is severe enough to produce a functional disability. **She has a history of a vertebral compression fracture 3 years ago after a fall in the bathroom.** Vertebral compression fracture in this age group implies the presence of osteopenia. One must also consider the possibility of metastatic tumor. The patient's history reveals at least two falling episodes. Therefore, consider etiologies for balance problems such as transient ischemic attacks or neuropathy.

PHYSICAL EXAMINATION

Physical examination reveals a frail elderly woman who is limping with a lurch over the right hip. She has a positive Trendelenburg's sign on the right (Fig 3.3). Limp

28

is a general term describing an abnormal gait. An antalgic gait is characterized by the patient spending less time on the involved leg. Lurching over the right hip, as well as the positive Trendelenburg's sign, reflects an involuntary attempt on the part of the patient to reduce the forces across the right hip. This is done by moving the center of gravity over the femoral head. **The range of motion of her hips is essentially symmetrical. However, the patient guards and has slight pain with internal rotation of her right hip.** These findings suggest some abnormality in the hip joint although they do not differentiate fracture from arthritis. **Percussion of either the right greater trochanter or the heel produces pain in the right groin.** Percussion pain implies bony discontinuity along the weight-bearing axis. **The patient cannot lift her right leg off the bed when her knee is extended.** Attempting to "straight leg raise" when the hip is fractured produces pain secondary to fracture motion from forces across the hip joint. **Alignment of both lower extremities appears normal.** When a hip fracture is displaced, the involved leg is shortened and externally rotated. The absence of this sign does not rule out the possibility of a broken hip.

LABORATORY FINDINGS

An AP x-ray of the affected hip is shown in Fig 3.4. The x-ray reveals an impacted intertrochanteric fracture in osteopenic bone and no radiographic evidence of tumor.

The patient should not be permitted to walk or bear weight on this leg. In addition, hip rotation and straight leg raising should be avoided.

29

4

Warm, Red, Swollen Knee

Warm, Red, Swollen Knee

Precipitating Event or Cause	Differential Diagnosis	Key Findings	Key Tests	Natural History if Untreated	Treatment	Expected Outcome with Treatment
Insidious (no overt event) Sudden Recent sexual contact or promiscuity History of gout Hereditary Occupational overuse	Gonorrheal septic arthritis	Skin lesions History of urethral discharge Migratory arthritis	Oral, rectal, vaginal/urethral cultures Gram stain Aspirate	Improvement	Penicillin	Normal joint
	RA	Polyarticular morning stiffness	RF adult ANA Synovial biopsy	Adults: variable progression	Aspirin NSAID Steroids Penicillin Gold	Variable progression Possible joint destruction
	Nongonorrheal septic arthritis pyogenic vs tubercular	Exquisitely painful range of motion	Joint fluid cell count and differential Glucose Gram stain Culture	Joint destruction	Drain Antibiotics	Resolution if treated early Joint destruction if treated late
	Gout Pseudogout	Exquisite tenderness	Joint fluid crystal analysis Serum uric acid Response to colchicine	Recurrence	NSAID Allopurinol Diet Colchicine	Tendency to recur May destroy joint

RA, rheumatoid arthritis; RF, rheumatoid factor; ANA, antinuclear antibodies; NSAID, nonsteroidal anti-inflammatory drugs.

Precipitating Event or Cause	Differential Diagnosis	Key Findings	Key Tests	Natural History if Untreated	Treatment	Expected Outcome with Treatment
Insidious (no overt event) Sudden Recent sexual contact or promiscuity History of gout Hereditary Occupational overuse	Bursitis (septic)	Swollen bursa No joint effusion Normal range of motion	Bursal aspirate Culture	Acute: resolution Chronic: recurrence	Splint NSAID Antibiotics if septic Excision if chronic	May recur Resolution
	Reiter's syndrome	History of urethral discharge Conjunctivitis	Culture positive for *Chlamydia*	Recurrence	Metronidazole (Flagyl) Tetracycline	Normal joint
	Cellulitis	Recent puncture, abrasion or laceration Streaking		Depends on organism	Antibiotics Moist, hot packs Elevation	Resolution

HISTORY

A 24-year-old white female divorcée presents with right knee pain and swelling of approximately 3 weeks' duration. She has noticed intermittent aching of other joints, a rash covering the trunk, and temperature elevation with sweats and chills over the past week. There has been no history of trauma or overuse.

PHYSICAL EXAMINATION

Examination reveals a female in moderate distress who limps and appears ill. Her temperature is 101°F. Her trunk is covered with a maculopapular rash. Her right knee is warm, has a moderate effusion, and is diffusely tender to palpation. Considerable pain occurs with passive range of motion. Knee ligaments are stable.

LABORATORY FINDINGS

X-rays of the knee (not shown) reveal an effusion. Under sterile conditions 50 ml of yellow opaque fluid are aspirated from the knee and sent to the laboratory for evaluation. The white blood cell count is 110,000. Seventy percent of the white cells are polymorphonuclear leukocytes. The aspirate glucose is lower than the blood glucose. No crystals are seen on microscopic evaluation. The Gram stain is negative for organisms. Cultures have been started but are not yet available.

QUESTIONS

1. What are the prognostic implications of a hot versus a cold swollen knee?
2. How do you decide whether this is a local or a systemic problem?
3. What arthritic problems are associated with rashes?

Discussion

HISTORY

A 24-year-old white female divorcée presents with right knee pain and swelling of approximately 3 weeks' duration. She has noticed intermittent aching of other joints, a rash covering the trunk, and temperature elevation with sweats and chills over the past week. A patient who has joint pain, swelling, and fever has a septic arthritis until proven otherwise. The problem began with knee swelling and later included systemic findings. Given the history of intermittent arthralgia, one must also consider migratory and polyarticular forms of arthritis. A rash associated with joint pain and fever is found in response to certain bacteria such as *Pneumococcus* or *Gonococcus*, with drug reactions, or in viral illnesses such as rubella. **There has been no history of trauma or overuse.** An internal knee derangement or tendinitis is unlikely.

Warm, Red, Swollen Knee

PHYSICAL EXAMINATION

Examination reveals a female in moderate distress who limps and appears ill. The process has both local and systemic manifestations. **Her temperature is 101°F.** This temperature is consistent with a bacterial or viral infection. **Her trunk is covered with a maculopapular rash.** The rash is another systemic manifestation. **Her right knee is warm, has a moderate effusion, and is diffusely tender to palpation.** This is an inflammatory rather than a mechanical process. The major concern in an inflamed joint is that it may be septic. Failure to treat a septic joint early can lead to joint destruction. **Considerable pain occurs with passive range of motion.** Cellulitis and bursitis about the knee are usually not aggravated by motion. **Knee ligaments are stable.** The ligaments have not been damaged by either trauma or long-standing inflammation.

LABORATORY FINDINGS

X-rays of the knee (not shown) reveal an effusion. Under sterile conditions 50 ml of yellow opaque fluid are aspirated from the knee and sent to the laboratory for evaluation. Opaque joint fluid is found in either inflamed or septic joints. Normal joint fluid is clear. **The white blood cell count is 110,000. Seventy percent of the white cells are polymorphonuclear leukocytes.** A white count this high with 70% PMNs is typical of septic arthritis. **The aspirate glucose is lower than the blood glucose.** Joint fluid glucose is much lower than blood glucose in the presence of a bacterial arthritis. **No crystals are seen on microscopic evaluation.** Gout and pseudogout are unlikely. **The Gram stain is negative for organisms.** The fact that no organisms are seen on Gram stain does not rule out infection. **Cultures have been started but are not yet available.**

HISTORY

The patient is a 34-year-old white female secretary who presents with a hot, red, swollen, painful left knee. The redness and pain began gradually 3 days ago, and symptoms have since progressed. She denies injury, recent sexual contact, drug abuse, or systemic infection. She is able to bear weight on the left leg. The knee is slightly painful with attempted motion. History is positive for intermittent bilateral wrist stiffness. She is taking no medication.

PHYSICAL EXAMINATION

The patient's temperature is 98.8°F. Her gait is antalgic, favoring the left leg. She has an obviously red, warm, swollen left knee. She has no skin lesions. No other joints appear abnormal. An effusion is present in the knee, and tenderness to palpation is quite diffuse. Knee range of motion from 10° to 70° causes minimal pain. There is no ligamentous laxity.

LABORATORY FINDINGS

Initial laboratory data include a hematocrit of 34 and a white blood cell count of 9,500.

QUESTIONS

1. Is the ability to bear weight on the involved extremity and move the knee consistent with its hot, red, swollen condition?
2. How do you distinguish between effusion, prepatellar bursitis, and cellulitis?
3. What other diagnostic studies might you perform at this time?
4. What is the single most important diagnostic test?

Discussion

HISTORY

The patient is a 34-year-old white female secretary who presents with a hot, red, swollen, painful left knee. The redness and pain began gradually 3 days ago, and symptoms have since progressed. Heat, redness, and swelling are signs of inflammation or sepsis. **She denies injury, recent sexual contact, drug abuse, or systemic infection.** Traumatic bursitis, synovitis secondary to a foreign body, gonorrhea, and sepsis from other pyogenic organisms are less likely. **She is able to bear weight on the left leg. The knee is slightly painful with attempted motion.** Inability to bear weight or move the knee is an indicator of severity. This knee is not severely involved with the disease process at this time. **History is positive for intermittent bilateral wrist stiffness.** Involvement of other joints suggests a systemic problem. **She is taking no medication.**

PHYSICAL EXAMINATION

The patient's temperature is 98.8°F. Her gait is antalgic, favoring the left leg. A septic joint is unlikely. **She has an obviously red, warm, swollen left knee.** These findings are typical of inflammatory arthritis. **She has no skin lesions.** Patients with gonococcal arthritis often have characteristic hemorrhagic vesicles or pustules with necrotic centers. Smears of these lesions found on the palms and fingers may reveal the gonococcus. **No other joints appear abnormal. An effusion is present in the knee, and tenderness to palpation is quite diffuse.** The presence of effusion differentiates intra-articular pathology from prepatellar bursitis or superficial cellulitis. **Knee range of motion from 10° to 70° causes minimal pain.** Moving a septic joint more than 5° to 10° produces exquisite pain. This patient's normal temperature and knee mobility are not consistent with sepsis. **There is no ligamentous laxity.**

LABORATORY FINDINGS

Initial laboratory data include a hematocrit of 34 and a white blood cell count of 9,500. The patient is slightly anemic and has a normal white count. These findings are not consistent with an acute inflammatory or septic process.

Other useful diagnostic studies include ESR, antinuclear antibodies, rheumatoid factor, serum uric acid, knee x-ray, and joint fluid analysis. Fluid should be analyzed for cell count and differential, crystals, and glucose, and should be sent for culture.

5   Leg Pain

Leg Pain

Precipitating Event or Cause	Differential Diagnosis	Key Findings	Key Tests	Natural History if Untreated	Treatment	Expected Outcome with Treatment
Increased activity Trauma Endogenous source of infection Insidious (no overt event)	Osteomyelitis	Point tenderness Fever History of upper respiratory or urinary tract infection	Needle aspirate for culture Bone scan	Sequestration	Drill Drainage Antibiotics	Early: cure Late: chronic drainage
	Fracture	Swelling Point tenderness Deformity	X-ray	Healing	Immobilize	Healing
	Stress fracture	Point tenderness History of increased activity Pain with excessive activity	Bone scan	Resolution	Decreased activity	Healing
	Chronic compartmental syndrome	History of numbness and pain with activity	Compartment pressures	Recurrence	Compartment release	Resolution
	Periostitis (shin splint)	Diffuse tenderness Pain with muscle use against resistance	Bone scan	Resolution	Ice Decreased activity NSAID	Resolution

NSAID, nonsteroidal anti-inflammatory drugs

Precipitating Event or Cause	Differential Diagnosis	Key Findings	Key Tests	Natural History if Untreated	Treatment	Expected Outcome with Treatment
Increased activity Trauma Endogenous source of infection Insidious (no overt event)	Tendinitis	History of increased activity Pain with use against resistance Crepitus over tendon sheath when tendon moves	None	Resolution	Rest NSAID Thermal modalities (ice, heat)	Resolution
	Tumor	Localized mass Pain	Biopsy	Progression	Excision or amputation Chemotherapy Radiation	Depends on tumor type
	Deep venous thrombosis	Swollen leg Calf pain Dilated veins Fever	Doppler exam Contrast phlebogram Isotopic venogram	Resolution or pulmonary embolus	Rest Elevation Anticoagulants	Early: resolution Late: chronic swelling

NSAID, nonsteroidal anti-inflammatory drugs

HISTORY

J.T. is a 6-year-old white boy who skidded while riding his bicycle and fell sideward. He is brought in by his mother 6 hours later becaue he refuses to walk. Past medical history is unremarkable.

PHYSICAL EXAMINATION

Physical examination reveals a charming little boy in mild distress who refuses to bear any weight on his right leg. The leg is minimally swollen, without redness or ecchymosis. There are no abrasions or lacerations on the lower extremity. The leg is tender to palpation over the middle to distal third of the tibia. The fibula, ankle, and knee are not tender to palpation. Sensation is intact over the areas of distribution of the superficial and deep peroneal nerves and the posterior tibial nerve. Motor function of the toes is normal. There is no pain with passive stretch of the toes.

LABORATORY FINDINGS

An AP x-ray of the patient's right tibia and fibula is shown in Fig 5.1.

QUESTIONS

1. What kinds of injuries would you suspect with this history?
2. What is the significance of a 6-year-old child's refusing to walk?
3. What principles guide the examination of a patient with possible fracture or ligamentous injury?

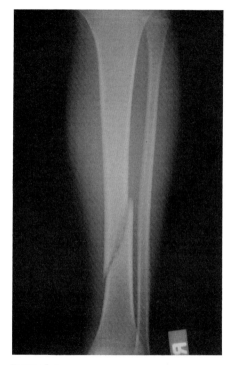

Figure 5.1

4. Why is the neurologic examination important in this setting?
5. Given the fracture pattern seen on x-ray, what is the likely mechanism of injury?

Discussion

HISTORY

J.T. is a 6-year-old white boy who skidded while riding his bicycle and fell sideward. This is relatively low-energy trauma and might cause a nondisplaced fracture, or a sprain of the knee or ankle. Epiphyseal injuries are more common than sprains in this age group. **He is brought in by his mother 6 hours later because he refuses to walk.** In a young child, refusal to walk is significant. Typical causes include fracture, septic lower extremity joint, and discitis. **Past medical history is unremarkable.** This tends to rule out chronic problems and particularly infection.

PHYSICAL EXAMINATION

Physical examination reveals a charming little boy in mild distress who refuses to bear any weight on his right leg. This implies significant injury to the right lower extremity but probably rules out discitis, as the patient will walk on the opposite leg. **The leg is minimally swollen, without redness or ecchymosis. There are no abrasions or lacerations on the lower extremity.** The lack of significant swelling after 6 hours suggests a low-energy injury. **The leg is tender to palpation over the middle to distal third of the tibia. The fibula, ankle, and knee are not tender to palpation.** The findings have now been localized to the middle to distal third of the tibia. The possibility of neoplasia with a coincidental injury has not been eliminated, however. **Sensation is intact over the areas of distribution of the superficial and deep peroneal nerves and the posterior tibial nerve. Motor function of the toes is normal. There is no pain with passive stretch of the toes.** It is important to document the neurological status at the time of initial examination to rule out neurological injury from the trauma. It is also important for future reference should any signs of compartmental syndrome arise.

The examination of a patient with a possible fracture or ligamentous injury should include notation of swelling and skin condition. One should note any deformity of the limb or any dysfunction such as refusal to bear weight. One should avoid severely stressing a limb that is point-tender, and one should splint the limb before sending the patient for x-rays if suspicious of a fracture.

LABORATORY FINDINGS

An AP x-ray of the patient's right tibia and fibula is shown in Fig 5.1. The x-ray reveals an oblique tibial fracture that is not displaced and thereby suggests a shear mechanism or probable twisting injury. There is no evidence of any periosteal reaction or osteopenia at the fracture site, making a pathologic fracture unlikely.

HISTORY

J.M. is a 15-year-old white female complaining of localized swelling in the right lower leg. Three months ago she had a minor fall but noted no swelling at that time. Two months before presenting she was participating in a track meet and began to notice swelling over the inside of her right lower leg. Her family physician thought this was a soft-tissue injury and applied an Ace wrap to her leg. She continued running until 2 weeks ago when, because of the persistence of the swelling, x-rays were taken. On the basis of the x-ray, her family physician thought she might have an infection, and she was treated with oral antibiotics for 1 week while resting in bed. The swelling remains and she now desires a second opinion. She denies pain, fever, chills, or significant weight loss. Additional past history is totally unremarkable.

PHYSICAL EXAMINATION

Physical examination reveals a healthy-appearing young female with no limp. She has no fever. She has obvious swelling in the distal medial part of the right lower extremity. This swollen area is not warm or red but is firm and slightly tender. There is no pain on percussing the heel. There is no adenopathy in the groin. Neurological examination and pulses are normal.

LABORATORY FINDINGS

Complete blood count and erythrocyte sedimentation rate are normal. X-rays obtained include an AP view of the right tibia and fibula (Fig 5.2, left) and a mortise view of the ankle (Fig 5.2, right).

QUESTIONS

1. What physical characteristics do you look for when examining a palpable extremity mass?
2. Develop a differential diagnosis and indicate the evidence for and against each diagnosis.
3. What other studies will help you make a diagnosis?

Discussion

HISTORY

J.M. is a 15-year-old white female complaining of localized swelling in the right lower leg. Three months ago she had a minor fall but noted no swelling at that time. Two months before presenting she was participating in a track meet and began to notice swelling over the inside of her right lower leg. Diagnoses we must consider include tumor, infection, and a healing stress fracture. Compartmental syndromes can produce swelling in the lower extremity; however, such swelling is usually diffuse. **Her family physician thought this was a soft-tissue injury and applied an Ace wrap to her leg.** Lack of pain makes an infection or stress fracture unlikely. **She continued running until 2 weeks ago when, because of the persistence of the swelling, x-rays were taken. On the basis of the x-ray, her family physician thought she**

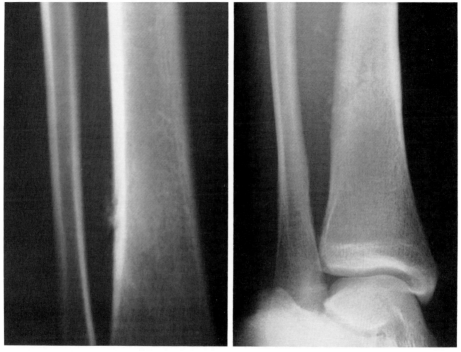

Figure 5.2

might have an infection, and she was treated with oral antibiotics for 1 week while resting in bed. The swelling remains and she now desires a second opinion. The persistence of swelling does not help us differentiate between the possible diagnoses. She denies pain, fever, chills, or significant weight loss. Additional history is totally unremarkable. The lack of pain makes fractures, tendinitis, or hematoma unlikely. Were infection responsible for the swelling, one would expect a history of pain, fever, and chills. Maintenance of weight suggests that the process has not become systemic.

PHYSICAL EXAMINATION

Physical examination reveals a healthy-appearing young female with no limp. Patients with significant tendinitis or fracture will splint the extremity by limping. She has no fever. A systemic illness is unlikely. She has obvious swelling in the distal medial part of the right lower extremity. This swollen area is not warm or red but is firm and slightly tender. When evaluating an extremity mass, one should observe skin color and the size and shape of the mass and look for dilation of surface blood vessels. On palpation, one should note whether there is increased skin temperature, tenderness, or ad-

herence of the mass to the skin. One should assess whether the mass is subcutaneous or deeper, fluctuant or firm, diffuse or well demarcated. In this patient, the lack of warmth, redness, or fluctuance makes infection unlikely. (We are not told whether the mass is fixed to the skin or is mobile. Malignancy must be suspected in adherent masses.) There is no pain on percussing the heel. Infection and fracture are unlikely. There is no adenopathy in the groin. Severe infection is unlikely. Neoplasia, if present, is not widespread. Neurologic examination and pulses are normal.

LABORATORY FINDINGS

Complete blood count and erythrocyte sedimentation rate are normal. These rule out a systemic illness. X-rays obtained include an AP view of the right tibia and fibula (Fig 5.2, left) and a mortise view of the ankle (Fig 5.2, right). The x-rays show calcific densities in the interosseous area. These make stress fracture unlikely and neoplasia or myositis ossificans more likely. The latter is usually associated with a clear history of injury.

Other helpful studies include MRI and arteriogram to determine the extent of local involvement; biopsy; and liver-spleen, lung, and bone scans to determine whether metastasis is present.

HISTORY

R.W. is a 9-year-old boy with a 7-day history of left knee pain. There is no previous history of injury, other joint pain, or rashes. The pain began insidiously. Five days prior to admission the patient had malaise, headache, nausea, and vomiting. Four days ago he developed a temperature of 103°F. The pain has become progressively worse since then.

PHYSICAL EXAMINATION

Physical examination reveals an ill-appearing child with a temperature of 100°F. The child walks with an antalgic gait favoring the left leg. He holds the left knee in a flexed position. There is no knee effusion, redness, or deformity. The knee is slightly warm to the touch and is tender at the medial and lateral tibial plateaus. Painless range of motion is from 60° to 120°. Attempts at straightening the knee beyond 60° of flexion are met with resistance due to pain.

LABORATORY FINDINGS

Laboratory data include a white blood cell count of 13,700 with 73% segmented polymorphonuclear leukocytes. ESR is 84 mm/h. One milliliter of fluid is aspirated from the knee. The fluid contains 9,700 white cells, 50% of which are PMNs. No bacteria are seen. An AP x-ray of the affected knee was obtained (Fig 5.3).

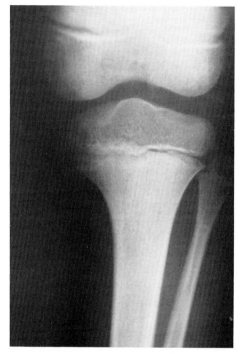

Figure 5.3

QUESTIONS

1. What evidence is there for systemic illness?
2. What are typical sources of referred pain to the knee in children?

3. Distinguish an antalgic gait from other gait abnormalities.
4. Of what significance are the lack of knee effusion and the painless 60° arc of motion?
5. Describe how the following are helpful:
   A. ESR and white blood cell count
   B. Joint fluid analysis
   C. X-ray
   D. Bone scan
6. What further tests would you perform?
7. If this represents an infectious process, what is the most likely causative organism?

Discussion

HISTORY

R.W. is a 9-year-old boy with a 7-day history of left knee pain. There is no previous history of injury, other joint pain, or rashes. It is unusual for a child to have a negative history for injury, but this certainly helps us rule out a knee fracture. In the pediatric age group, a slipped capital femoral epiphysis or Legg-Calvé-Perthes disease may present as knee pain referred from the hip. The lack of other joint pain or rashes makes rheumatic fever less likely. Some forms of juvenile rheumatoid arthritis can present in this way. **The pain began insidiously. Five days prior to admission the patient had malaise, headache, nausea, and vomiting.** This suggests a systemic problem and makes the hip diseases mentioned above less likely. **Four days ago he developed a temperature of 103°F. The pain has become progressively worse since then.** We have more evidence for a systemic problem such as infection, juvenile rheumatoid arthritis, or possibly a malignant neoplasm such as a Ewing's sarcoma.

PHYSICAL EXAMINATION

Physical examination reveals an ill-appearing child with a temperature of 100°F. This validates our impression above. **The child walks with an antalgic gait favoring the left leg.** An antalgic gait is manifested by decreased stance phase on the involved limb compared to the opposite limb. Patients often unconsciously adopt this gait because it decreases forces on and therefore pain in the involved limb. **He holds the left knee in a flexed position. There is no knee effusion, redness, or deformity.** The lack of knee effusion makes inflammatory or infectious arthritis less likely than a neighboring osteomyelitis or neoplasia. **The knee is slightly warm to the touch and is tender at the medial and lateral tibial plateaus.** These localized findings rule out referred pain. **Painless range of motion is from 60° to 120°. Attempts at straightening the knee beyond 60° of flexion are met with resistance due to pain.** A septic joint generally has an exquisitely painful and markedly limited range of motion; i.e., the patient will not allow any range of motion of the joint. Hence, this degree of painless motion confirms impressions that an osteomyelitis or neoplastic process near the knee is more likely.

LABORATORY FINDINGS

Laboratory examination includes a white blood cell count of 13,700 with 73% segmented polymorphonuclear leukocytes. ESR is 84 mm/h. The elevated white count and elevated percentage of polymorphonuclear leukocytes as well as an ESR rate of 84 suggest either an infectious process or a malignant neoplastic process, most commonly Ewing's sarcoma in this age group. **One milliliter of fluid is aspirated from the knee. The fluid contains 9,700 white cells, 50% of which are PMNs. No bacteria are seen.** In septic joints one would expect a much larger effusion with more white cells and a higher percentage of PMNs. It is not uncommon for an osteomyelitis near a joint to produce a sympathetic effusion in that joint. This effusion is in response to an irritated bony focus nearby and generally has a white count under 20,000 and fewer than 75% PMNs. Inflammatory joints (e.g., rheumatoid arthritis) have between 20,000 and 100,000 cells, whereas infected joints usually have greater than 100,000 cells and greater than 75% PMNs.

An AP x-ray of the affected knee was obtained (Fig 5.3). The x-ray reveals lytic areas in the medial tibial epiphysis and metaphysis. Infections are more likely to cross the physis than are tumors. The fact that there is no periosteal elevation does not eliminate osteomyelitis in its early stages. The organism that most commonly causes osteomyelitis in this age group is *Staphylococcus aureus*. Bone scan will not differentiate infection or inflammation from tumor. A needle biopsy for histology and culture would be useful.

HISTORY

The patient is a 19-year-old female who comes in complaining of bilateral "shin splints." She has had pain for 5 months in the anterior tibial areas of both legs. Five months ago she was playing racquetball as well as doing aerobic dancing and was working out 5 days a week. In her right leg, the pain would begin at the start of each aerobics class or racquetball game and was relieved by sitting or lying down. In her left leg, the pain was noticeable toward the end of a class or game and persisted for a few days after each activity. Because of the daily nature of her activities she has had pain on a daily basis, even while walking. The pain did not wake her from sleep. She has noted no swelling or numbness in either leg or foot. Three months ago the patient stopped exercising and was relieved of pain after a 2-week rest. She then returned to activity and had a recurrence of the same problem. She has been off all exercise for the last 6 weeks and says that the symptoms have improved in that now she can walk without pain.

PHYSICAL EXAMINATION

On physical examination the patient has a normal gait and no obvious swelling or masses in either leg. Her left leg is tender along the medial border of the tibia in its middle third for a distance of about 6 inches. Her right tibia is tender over a 1-inch area at the medial border of its distal third. She has no pain in either leg with use of the posterior or anterior tibial muscles against resistance. Her feet are quite pronated bilaterally. Pounding on the patient's heels in line with the axis of the tibia produces pain in the right leg only.

LABORATORY FINDINGS

Bone scans of both legs were obtained (Fig 5.4, left leg on left).

QUESTIONS

1. What types of conditions can present as "shin splints"?
2. How do you distinguish between the various diagnostic possibilities by either history or physical examination?
3. Why did the patient develop this particular problem at this particular time?

Discussion

HISTORY

The patient is a 19-year-old female who comes in complaining of bilateral "shin splints." Shin splints, or pain at the anterior border of the tibia, can represent a stress fracture of the tibia, a muscle strain of the anterior or posterior tibial muscles at their origins, or a chronic compartmental syndrome. **She has had pain for 5 months in the anterior tibial areas of both legs.** The duration rules out an acute fracture; the bilaterality makes a tumor less likely. **Five months ago she was playing racquetball as well as doing aerobic dancing and was working out 5**

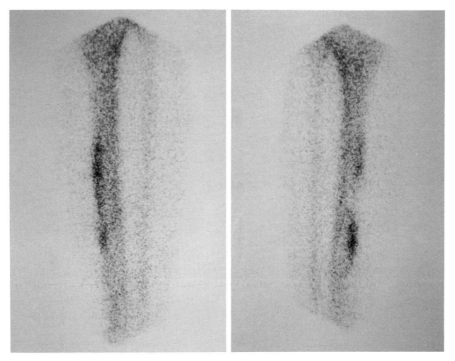

Figure 5.4

days a week. The intensity of activity makes overuse problems likely. **In her right leg, the pain would begin at the start of each aerobics class or racquetball game and was relieved by sitting or lying down.** Pain that begins immediately upon impact and is relieved by avoiding weight bearing is consistent with a stress fracture. **In her left leg, the pain was noticeable toward the end of a class or game and persisted for a few days after each activity.** This pain is consistent with a muscle strain (periostitis). Pain due to compartmental syndrome is more likely to come on during an activity, because of the swelling in the limb at that time, but resolve within a few hours. **Because of the daily nature of her activities she has had pain on a daily basis even while walking.** The patient never rested enough to relieve either leg of its problem. **The pain did not wake her from sleep.** This supports the impression that a tumor is unlikely. **She has noted no swelling or numbness in either leg or foot.** Swelling or numbness occasionally is found in a patient with a chronic compartmental syndrome. The numbness is characteristically found in the distribution of the involved peripheral nerve. **Three months ago the patient stopped exercising and was relieved of pain after a 2-week rest. She then returned to activity and had a recurrence of the same problem.** This information confirms the likely overuse origin. **She has been off all exercise for the last 6 weeks and says that the symptoms have improved in that now she can walk without pain.** Both processes are resolving somewhat with rest.

PHYSICAL EXAMINATION

On physical examination the patient has a normal gait and no obvious swelling or masses in either leg. The problems are not acute. Occasionally patients with a compartmental syndrome will have a small muscular hernia that is noted when standing. In addition, a healing stress fracture may produce a small lump on the tibia; a very active chronic periostitis may produce a ridge on the anterior tibia. **Her left leg is tender along the medial border of the tibia in its middle third for a distance of about 6 inches.** Compartmental syndromes usually present without any tenderness unless the patient has exercised immediately prior to examination. The extent of the tenderness is more consistent with an inflammation at the muscle attachment rather than a single stress fracture. **Her right tibia is tender over a 1-inch area at the medial border of its distal third.** This localized tenderness is consistent with a stress fracture. **She has no pain in either leg with use of the posterior or anterior tibial muscles against resistance.** Often muscular strain or periostitis will produce pain with use of involved muscles against resistance. However, this patient has not exercised for 6 weeks, and the process is less acute. Stress fractures and compartmental syndromes should not produce pain with use of muscles against resistance. **Her feet are quite pronated bilaterally.** Pronated feet increase tension on the posterior tibial musculotendinous unit with each step and can lead to periostitis. **Pounding on**

the patient's heels in line with the axis of the tibia produces pain in the right leg only. Impact pain is consistent with a stress fracture and mimics what the patient does when she jumps or runs on that leg.

LABORATORY FINDINGS

Bone scans of both legs were obtained (Fig 5.4, left leg on left). On both legs, the bone scan reveals areas of increased uptake, which correspond to the sites of tenderness. The bone scan of the left leg reveals increased uptake diffusely along the anteromedial aspect of the tibia. This is consistent with periostitis. On the right leg, the increased uptake is very well localized to a small area. This is consistent with a stress fracture.

6   Ankle Pain

Ankle Pain

Precipitating Event or Cause	Differential Diagnosis	Key Findings	Key Tests	Natural History if Untreated	Treatment	Expected Outcome with Treatment

Twisting episode
Recent change in activity
Unusual activity
  Occupation
  Sport
Endogenous infection
Insidious (no overt event)
	Sprain	History of trauma
		Localized tenderness and swelling (early)
			Stress films	Mild: healing	Rest, ice, compression, elevation, "RICE"	Mild: normal ankle

				Severe: chronic instability and DJD	Cast vs operative repair	Severe: slightly decreased range of motion, some instability
	Tendinitis (anterior or posterior tibial, peroneal, Achilles)	Pain with use against resistance Crepitus with movement Increased local heat	None	Gradual resolution	Rest Thermal modalities (ice, heat) Ultrasound NSAID	Resolution Possible recurrence
	Stress fracture (distal fibula or tibia)	History of increased activity Local tenderness Increased warmth Impulse pain	Bone scan x-rays	Complete fracture if not restricted	Restrict activity	Healing
	Ankle DJD	Pain increased with activity Barometric sensitivity Chronicity	Ankle x-ray	Progression Decreased range of motion	NSAID Rest Support (brace, crutches, orthotics)	Progressive functional limitations

NSAID, nonsteroidal anti-inflammatory drugs; DJD, degenerative joint disease.

Precipitating Event or Cause	Differential Diagnosis	Key Findings	Key Tests	Natural History if Untreated	Treatment	Expected Outcome with Treatment
Twisting episode Recent activity change Unusual activity Occupation Sport Endogenous infection Insidious (no overt event)	Subtalar DJD	Previous fracture involving subtalar joint History of severe sprain Pain when walking on uneven ground Pain on inversion and eversion or standing, referred to inframalleolar region	Subtalar joint x-ray	Progression Decreased range of motion	NSAID Rest Support (brace, crutches, orthotics)	Progressive functional limitations
	Inflammatory arthritis Reiter's syndrome RA	Polyarticular involvement History of systemic arthritis	Synovial biopsy	Recurrence	NSAID Rest Synovectomy	Recurrence Progressive functional limitations
	Infectious arthritis	Infection elsewhere Local puncture Exquisitely painful Patient refuses joint motion	Culture of joint fluid	Progressive joint destruction	Drainage Antibiotics Immobilization	Early: complete resolution Late: functional limitation
	Osteochondral defects: Osteochondritis dissecans Loose body	History of trauma Aching pain Catching Effusion	Arthrotomograms	Chronic synovitis DJD	Drilling and/or excision	Occasional pain and stiffness

DJD, degenerative joint disease; RA, rheumatoid arthritis; NSAID, nonsteroidal anti-inflammatory drugs.

HISTORY

This 25-year-old graduate student in psychology presents with a 2-year history of chronic left ankle instability. While playing a variety of collegiate sports, the patient experienced multiple left ankle sprains, none of which was treated by a physician. Over the past 2 years the tendency for inversion sprains of the left ankle has increased, with a frequency of about one every 3 months. Initially these episodes were precipitated by walking on uneven ground, but now they occur on level ground without predictability. The patient feels particularly susceptible when descending stairs or when trying to turn or stop suddenly while running. After each episode the ankle swells and aches for a week and then returns to its present state.

PHYSICAL EXAMINATION

Physical examination shows a healthy-appearing male with normal lower extremity alignment. Swelling and thickening of the tissues are evident around the anterior aspect of the left ankle joint. Range of motion in both the tibiotalar and subtalar joints is normal bilaterally. The patient walks without a limp. When the left foot is passively twisted into maximal inversion, the lateral border of the talus can be felt laterally just anterior to the tip of the fibula. This finding is not present in the right ankle.

LABORATORY FINDINGS

Fig 6.1 shows an AP radiograph of both ankles during stress testing (left) and lateral views of the left ankle during anterior drawer stress testing (center and right).

QUESTIONS

1. Are there indications of articular surface damage or the presence of a loose body?
2. What conditions can cause these symptoms and how are they diagnosed?
3. What factors are important in ankle stability?
4. Explain the pathomechanics of instability while descending stairs or stopping suddenly.
5. Why has this patient's problem persisted?

Discussion

HISTORY

This 25-year-old graduate student in psychology presents with a 2-year history of chronic left ankle instability. While playing a variety of collegiate sports, the patient experienced multiple left ankle sprains, none of which was treated by a physician. The patient's sprains were not properly protected, and the ligaments have healed in a lengthened position. The condition has become chronic because of permanent damage to the ligamentous integrity. **Over the past 2 years the tendency for inversion sprains of the left ankle has increased,**

58

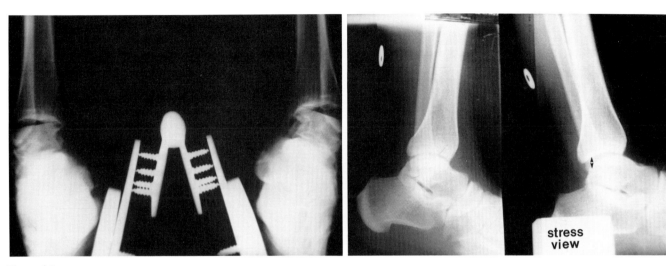

Figure 6.1

with a frequency of about one every 3 months. Initially these episodes were precipitated by walking on uneven ground, but now they occur on level ground without predictability. With each additional inversion injury, further elongation of the already-damaged ligaments takes place making the ankle less stable and easier to reinjure. In addition, loss of the proprioceptive input from normal ligaments makes the ankle harder to control muscularly. The patient feels particularly susceptible when descending stairs or trying to turn or stop suddenly while running. This is caused by abnormal shifting of the talus in the ankle mortise. After each episode the ankle swells and aches for a week and then returns to its present state. This suggests further injury of the ligaments and potentially of the articular surfaces of the ankle.

PHYSICAL EXAMINATION

Physical examination shows a healthy-appearing male with normal lower extremity alignment. There is no obvious anatomic abnormality such as genu varum or

59

hindfoot varus, which might predispose this patient to recurrent inversion injuries. **Swelling and thickening of the tissues are evident around the anterior aspect of the left ankle joint.** Ankle effusions most commonly present anterolaterally and reflect irritation in the ankle joint. In this setting, irritation could be secondary to instability or a loose body. **Range of motion in both the tibiotalar and subtalar joints is normal bilaterally.** This suggests that arthritic changes have not taken place and that the problem is not one of tarsal coalition in the subtalar or midfoot joints. **The patient walks without a limp.** Presently he is in no pain. **When the left foot is passively twisted into maximal inversion, the lateral border of the talus can be felt laterally just anterior to the tip of the fibula. This finding is not present in the right ankle.** Clinically appreciable talar tilt, if unilateral, is a reliable sign of insufficiency of the calcaneofibular ligament. There is a wide range of normal in talar tilt, and one should always compare the affected side with the normal side.

LABORATORY FINDINGS

Fig 6.1 shows an AP radiograph of both ankles during stress testing (left) and lateral radiographs of the left ankle during anterior drawer stress testing (center and right). Stress films reveal excessive talar tilt as well as abnormal anterior mobility of the talus (anterior drawer). Excessive talar tilt indicates insufficiency of the calcaneofibular ligament, whereas excessive anterior drawer indicates insufficiency of the anterior talofibular ligament. Stress films are required to assess ankle laxity objectively. An arthrogram would reveal loose bodies if present.

HISTORY

I.B. is a 28-year-old professional ballet dancer who complains of medial arch pain, especially when her foot is pointed in a plantarflexed position. This pain began 1 month ago when, in addition to her usual classwork, she rehearsed 4 to 5 hours per day for an upcoming performance. There has been no ecchymosis or swelling. The problem has not responded to a 2-week course of anti-inflammatory drugs.

PHYSICAL EXAMINATION

On physical examination the patient's gait is normal. No warmth, swelling, or tenderness is present around the Achilles tendon. However, swelling and slight tenderness are noted posterior to the medial malleolus, extending distally to the level of the tarsometatarsal joint. Inversion and plantarflexion of the foot against resistance cause medial arch pain. Crepitus is noted behind the medial malleolus during active ankle motion.

QUESTIONS

1. What conditions can cause these symptoms?
2. What might produce this type of problem?
3. What anatomic factors contribute to this type of problem?
4. Why has this problem developed at this particular time in this dancer's career?
5. What are the pathomechanics of the crepitus noted behind the medial malleolus?
6. What is the value of the test in which the patient resists inversion and plantarflexion of the foot?

Discussion

HISTORY

I.B. is a 28-year-old professional ballet dancer who complains of medial arch pain, especially when her foot is pointed in a plantarflexed position. The localization of pain to this area suggests involvement of the posterior tibial tendon, the plantar fascia, or neurologic structures in the tarsal tunnel. These structures may be affected by tendinitis, fasciitis, or nerve entrapment, respectively. **This pain began 1 month ago when, in addition to her usual classwork, she rehearsed 4 to 5 hours per day for an upcoming performance.** This history suggests that overuse may have contributed to the problem. **There has been no ecchymosis or swelling.** Trauma does not seem to be a contributing factor. Other causative factors to consider include underlying metabolic problems, anatomic anomalies, and previous injury. **The problem has not responded to a 2-week course of anti-inflammatory drugs.** This lack of response does not necessarily rule out an inflammatory process, particularly if the patient has continued to overuse the involved foot.

PHYSICAL EXAMINATION

On physical examination the patient's gait is normal. This suggests that the structure involved is not painful 61

Ankle Pain

Case 11. 28-Year-Old Professional Dancer

during normal gait. **No warmth, swelling, or tenderness is present around the Achilles tendon. However, swelling and slight tenderness are noted posterior to the medial malleolus, extending distally to the level of the tarsometatarsal joint.** The swelling and tenderness in this area eliminate the plantar fascia as a source of the problem and incriminate structures that pass posterior to the medial malleolus and extend distally to the tarsometatarsal joint. These structures include the posterior tibial neurovascular bundle, the tibialis posterior tendon, the flexor hallucis tendon, and the flexor digitorum longus tendon. **Inversion and plantarflexion of the foot against resistance cause medial arch pain.** This motion specifi-

cally tests the posterior tibial tendon and hence suggests it as the source of pain rather than the other structures noted above. **Crepitus is noted behind the medial malleolus during active ankle motion.** Crepitus usually suggests inflammation of the structures within the tendon sheath. This, in combination with the pain during resisted inversion and plantarflexion of the foot, suggests a tenosynovitis of the posterior tibial tendon. This inflammation most likely has developed at this time because of overuse while rehearsing. Anatomic factors that contribute to this type of problem include hypermobility, pronation, tight Achilles tendon, and excessive heel valgus.

62

HISTORY

This 32-year-old male office worker complains of left ankle pain and swelling, which have persisted for 3 months. Three months ago while hiking, he twisted his left ankle. He experienced pain and noted immediate swelling about the ankle but was able to return to his car unaided. He went to a hospital emergency room for evaluation and was told that he had torn the medial ligament of his ankle. His ankle was casted for 6 weeks, during which time he was able to bear weight without pain. Several days after removal of the cast the ankle again became painful. Treatment at that time consisted of active assisted exercises to restore ankle motion. The ankle has remained stiff and painful.

PHYSICAL EXAMINATION

Examination shows a healthy male in no distress, with pertinent findings limited to the left ankle. The patient walks with a left-sided antalgic gait. Moderate swelling is present about the anterolateral aspect of the ankle. There is tenderness to palpation about the anteromedial joint line. Plantarflexion is normal. The left ankle cannot be dorsiflexed beyond neutral whereas the right ankle dorsiflexes 20°. The left subtalar joint moves through a 10° arc of motion whereas the right moves through 35°. Stress testing in the anterior-posterior, medial-lateral, and inversion-eversion directions shows no increased laxity.

LABORATORY FINDINGS

A mortise view of the left ankle was obtained (Fig 6.2).

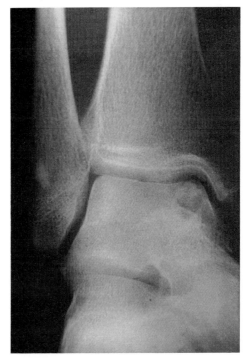

Figure 6.2

QUESTIONS

1. What are the possible causes for decreased ankle motion on physical examination?
2. Given persistent symptoms in a patient who appeared to have a simple ankle sprain, how would your workup proceed?

Discussion

HISTORY

This 32-year-old male office worker complains of left ankle pain and swelling, which have persisted for 3 months. Three months ago while hiking, he twisted his left ankle. Uncomplicated sprains usually heal in 6 to 8 weeks. **He experienced pain and noted immediate swelling about the ankle but was able to return to his car unaided.** Fractures and major ligamentous injury are unlikely. **He went to a hospital emergency room for evaluation and was told he had torn the medial ligament of his ankle.** This is probably the deltoid ligament. **His ankle was casted for 6 weeks, during which time he was able to bear weight without pain.** Ankle sprains can be protected while healing either in plaster or by weight bearing as tolerated on crutches. Casting provides a more stable environment for healing but leads to joint stiffness. Treatment without plaster but with a compression wrap to control swelling helps to retain ankle motion and muscle function. Fractures or gross instability require

cast protection and often surgical intervention. **Several days after removal of the cast the ankle again became painful.** Pain is an unexpected finding given the symptomatic relief in plaster. It suggests incomplete healing or that another problem exists. **Treatment at that time consisted of active assisted exercises to restore ankle motion.** Physical therapy is the appropriate treatment for regaining normal motion after a period of immobilization. **The ankle has remained stiff and painful.** Persistent stiffness, swelling, and pain 3 months after the injury raise the question of other problems in the ankle joint.

PHYSICAL EXAMINATION

Examination shows a healthy male in no distress, with pertinent findings limited to the left ankle. The patient walks with a left-sided antalgic gait. The left ankle is painful. **Moderate swelling is present about the anterolateral aspect of the ankle.** This is the usual location for swelling from within the ankle joint. **There is tenderness to palpation about the anteromedial joint line.** Tenderness in this area suggests an incompletely healed deltoid ligament, loose bodies, or fracture of the anteromedial corner of the talus. **Plantarflexion is normal. The left ankle cannot be dorsiflexed beyond neutral whereas the right ankle dorsiflexes 20°. The left subtalar joint moves through a 10° arc of motion whereas the right moves through 35°.** These findings are consistent with a prolonged period of immobilization and inadequate rehabilitation. Decreased motion can also be due to patient resistance, tight heel cords, bony spurs, loose bodies, joint adhesions or joint incongruity. **Stress testing in the anterior-posterior, medial-lateral, and inversion-eversion directions shows no increased laxity.** Stress testing involves forceful manipulation of the ankle joint; one looks for increased laxity of the talus within the ankle mortise. Mortise laxity can also be demonstrated radiographically using stress films.

LABORATORY FINDINGS

A mortise view of the ankle was obtained (Fig 6.2). The x-ray reveals an abnormality in the anteromedial corner of the talus, consistent with an osteochondral fracture or osteochondritis dissecans. In similar clinical settings in which the plain film is normal, arthrography or CT scanning can be helpful in revealing a chondral fracture or smaller osteochondral fracture.

Ankle Pain

HISTORY

The patient is a 50-year-old female who complains of left ankle pain of 1 year's duration. Five years ago she fell while mountain climbing, sustaining a minimally displaced lateral malleolar fracture. This was treated nonoperatively in plaster for 6 weeks. The patient did well until 1 year ago. At that time she noted a gradual onset of aching pain, which is aggravated by bearing weight and by movement at the ankle. The pain is also worse during inclement weather. Her occupation as a museum docent requires that she stand and walk on marble floors for 5 to 6 hours a day. Her family physician prescribed ibuprofen (Motrin) 400 mg q.i.d., which has helped but has not completely relieved the nagging ache.

PHYSICAL EXAMINATION

Physical examination reveals a healthy-appearing female who is slightly overweight and who walks with an antalgic gait favoring the left leg. She is wearing medium-heeled shoes. The limp increases when she is walking barefoot. When the patient is sitting, her left ankle appears somewhat swollen and is warmer to touch than the opposite ankle. Palpation about the ankle joint reveals tenderness and thickening anteriorly. Passive range of motion examination reveals the following:

	Right	Left
Dorsiflexion from neutral	30°	0°
Plantarflexion from neutral	20°	15°
Subtalar inversion	10°	10°
Subtalar eversion	5°	5°
Forefoot motion	Supple	Supple

LABORATORY FINDINGS

Fig 6.3 shows an AP radiograph of both ankles.

QUESTIONS

1. What is the relationship of the fracture to the patient's present problem?

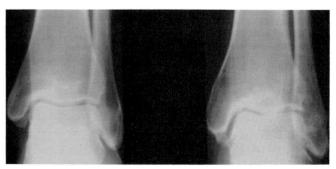

Figure 6.3

66

2. Compare and contrast the patient's problem with that of inflammatory arthritis involving the foot and ankle.
3. Why is the limp worse without shoes than with shoes?

Discussion

HISTORY

The patient is a 50-year-old female who complains of left ankle pain of 1 year's duration. This suggests a chronic condition. **Five years ago she fell while mountain climbing, sustaining a minimally displaced lateral malleolar fracture.** Intra-articular ankle fractures may produce incongruity of the articular surfaces, necrosis of articular cartilage, loose bodies, or abnormal biomechanics of the joint. **This was treated nonoperatively in plaster for 6 weeks.** Nonoperative treatment of minimally displaced fractures is acceptable. **The patient did well until 1 year ago. At that time she noted a gradual onset of aching pain, which is aggravated by bearing weight and by movement at the ankle.** Inflammatory arthritis produces pain independent of weight bearing. A loose body or osteochondritis dissecans is less likely given the length of the asymptomatic interval. **The pain is also worse during inclement weather.** Symptoms of degenerative arthritis are aggravated by drops in barometric pressure. These pressure changes do not affect inflammatory arthritis. **Her occupation as a museum docent requires that she stand and walk on marble floors for 5 to 6 hours a day.** Standing and walking for long periods on hard floors are poorly tolerated by arthritic joints whose articular surfaces have lost their inherent shock-absorbing capacity. **Her family physician prescribed ibuprofen (Motrin) 400 q.i.d., which has helped but has not competely relieved the nagging ache.** Inflammation is only one component of the patient's problem.

PHYSICAL EXAMINATION

Physical examination reveals a healthy-appearing female who is slightly overweight and who walks with an antalgic gait favoring the left leg. Obesity increases forces across weight-bearing joints. The antalgic gait reflects the patient's desire to minimize weight-bearing time on the affected leg. **She is wearing medium-heeled shoes. The limp increases when she is walking barefoot.** Shoes provide shock absorption. Medium-height heels minimize the ankle motion required during walking. **When the patient is sitting, her left ankle appears somewhat swollen and is warmer to touch than the opposite ankle.** Swelling and warmth are consistent with either an inflammatory or a degenerative joint problem. **Palpation about the ankle joint reveals tenderness and thickening anteriorly.** Soft-tissue thickening suggests that this condition has become chronic. **Passive range of motion examination reveals the following:** (See range of motion chart.) Left ankle motion is restricted. The subtalar joint is unaffected. Degenerative joint disease causes hypertrophic spurring about the joint margins and loss of joint space, both of which tend to limit motion. Although

67

degenerative joint disease may be secondary to inflammatory arthritis, this patient's picture is most consistent with posttraumatic degenerative joint disease of the ankle, probably the result of joint incongruity related to her fracture 5 years earlier.

LABORATORY FINDINGS

Fig 6.3 shows an AP radiograph of both ankles. The x-ray reveals early degenerative joint disease of the left ankle as manifested by increased sclerosis in the tibial plafond as well as osteophyte formation medially.

7

Foot Pain

Foot Pain

Precipitating Event or Cause	Differential Diagnosis	Key Findings	Key Tests	Natural History if Untreated	Treatment	Expected Outcome with Treatment
Poorly fitting shoes Excessive or unusual activity Localized weight concentration on one or more metatarsal heads Old injury Neuromuscular imbalance Hereditary Insidious (no overt event)	Morton's neuroma	Third web space numbness Pain radiating into third and fourth toes reproduced by medial-lateral compression or plantar axial pressure between third and fourth metatarsal heads	Pain relieved by intermetatarsal nerve block	Variable	Acute: metatarsal pad Chronic: steroid injection Excision of neuroma	Pain relief Residual numbness in third web space
	Metatarsalgia	Pain under the metatarsal head(s) Abnormally distributed callosities Poor plantar pad thickness Cavus foot	X-rays	Persistence	Metatarsal pads and bars If rheumatoid: resection of metatarsal heads	Pain relief
	Gout	Inflamed first MTP joint Exquisite pain	Aspirate MTP joint for crystals Serum uric acid Response to colchicine	Recurrence	Acute: NSAID Colchicine Chronic: Dietary change Allopurinol	Resolution of acute attack Tendency to recur May destroy joint
	Hallux valgus	Metatarsus primus varus Painful bunion Pronated foot	X-rays while bearing weight	Progressive MTP joint DJD	Shoes with adequate width Arch supports to reduce pronation	Dependent on severity
					Realignment and removal of bunion	Correction of deformity and pain relief

MTP, metatarsophalangeal; NSAID, nonsteroidal anti-inflammatory drugs; DJD, degenerative joint disease.

Foot Pain

Precipitating Event or Cause	Differential Diagnosis	Key Findings	Key Tests	Natural History if Untreated	Treatment	Expected Outcome with Treatment
Poorly fitting shoes Excessive or unusual activity Localized weight concentration to one or more metatarsal heads Old injury Neuromuscular imbalance Hereditary Insidious (no overt event)	Hammer toes	PIP joint flexion contracture Callus over dorsal PIP joint and tip of distal phalanx	X-ray	Persistent pain and deformity	Resection of PIP joint with optional fusion	Pain relief
	Claw toes	MTP hyperextension PIP and DIP flexion Toes may not contact floor Deformity may be static or dynamic	X-ray	May lead to metatarsalgia and callosities	Metatarsal pad or bar Tendon release/balance	Symptomatic relief
	Hallux rigidus (DJD of the first MTP joint)	Long first ray Decreased first MTP motion, especially dorsiflexion	X-ray	Progression	Fusion of the MTP joint in 30° of dorsiflexion or Silastic joint replacement	Pain relief
	Freiberg's infraction (AVN of second metatarsal head)	Pain and dorsal swelling over second MTP joint	X-ray	Pain and decreased motion of joint	Nonoperative: metatarsal relief pad	Pain relief
					Operative: resection of base of second proximal phalanx	Pain relief

PIP, proximal interphalangeal; DIP, distal interphalangeal; MTP, metatarsophalangeal; DJD, degenerative joint disease; AVN, avascular necrosis.

Foot Pain

Precipitating Event or Cause	Differential Diagnosis	Key Findings	Key Tests	Natural History if Untreated	Treatment	Expected Outcome with Treatment
Poorly fitting shoes Excessive or unusual activity Localized weight concentration on one or more metatarsal heads Old injury Neuromuscular imbalance Hereditary Insidious (no overt event)	Neuropathy (alcoholic, diabetic)	Burning sensation in feet	Nerve conduction velocity	Persistence	Control hypoglycemia Vitamin B_{12} injections	Variable
	Plantar fasciitis (heel spur)	Pronated foot Tenderness at fascial origin Cavus foot	None	Persistent	Orthotics to support medial arch NSAID Tape Steroid injection	Tendency to recur
	Seronegative spondyloarthropathies	Chest expansion less than 2 inches	HLA-B-27	Recurrence	NSAID	Intermittent flares
	Stress fracture	Local tenderness	Bone scan	Healing	Decreased activity Stiff-soled shoe or cast	Healing

NSAID, nonsteroidal anti-inflammatory drugs.

HISTORY

A 26-year-old female university dance student presents with well-localized, nonradiating pain on the dorsum of her left foot. The pain began 2 months ago. Before then she had been taking 4 hours of dance classes per week. When school began again 2 months ago, the number of class hours increased to 20 per week. In class she was required to jump frequently. The onset of pain in her foot was quite abrupt and prevented her from putting weight on the foot for 1 week. Although pain prevented her from dancing for 2 additional weeks, she could walk during that time. She then began dancing again and noted that, compared to previously, the pain in her foot had decreased but the swelling had increased.

PHYSICAL EXAMINATION

Physical examination reveals a normal gait. The patient has localized swelling in the area of the third metatarsal. In addition, this area is tender to palpation, particularly in the area of the third metatarsal neck. Lateral compression of the metatarsals is not painful. Sensory examination is normal.

LABORATORY FINDINGS

AP and oblique x-rays taken shortly after the onset of pain are presented at left in Fig 7.1. AP and oblique views taken at the time of presentation 2 months later are shown at right in the figure.

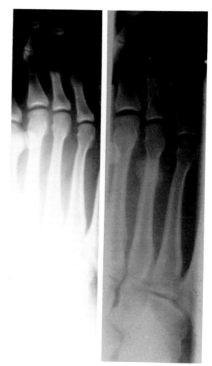

Figure 7.1

QUESTIONS

1. Why has this problem developed at this particular time?
2. Explain the increased swelling accompanied by decreased pain.
3. Is this an acute problem getting better or the onset of a chronic problem?
4. What are you trying to elicit when you compress metatarsals laterally as opposed to compressing them individually in the anteroposterior plane?

Discussion

HISTORY

A 26-year-old female university dance student presents with well-localized, nonradiating pain on the dorsum of her left foot. The pain began 2 months ago. The duration of the pain suggests that the problem currently is not one of acute trauma, and its nonradiating character makes referred or neural problems less likely. The dorsum of the foot is a common place for presentation of pain from bony lesions in the foot as well as from extensor tendon inflammation. **Before then she had been taking 4 hours of dance classes per week. When school began again 2 months ago, the number of class hours increased to 20 per week.** The history of a recent increase in activity often suggests an overuse problem. **In class she was required to jump frequently.** This also provides the set-

ting for an overuse injury. **The onset of pain in her foot was quite abrupt and prevented her from putting weight on the foot for 1 week.** The abrupt onset suggests that a traumatic injury occurred at that time. One should be able to bear weight with tendinitis; hence, this history indicates a bony lesion as the source of pain. **Although pain prevented her from dancing for 2 additional weeks, she could walk during that time.** The amount of weight that can be borne is a measure of the severity of the problem. **She then began dancing again and noted that, compared to previously, the pain in her foot had decreased but the swelling had increased.** In most inflammatory processes, including tendinitis or a neuroma, the swelling increases as the pain increases. In this case, the increased swelling may represent a healing process, which explains why the pain can decrease at the same time.

PHYSICAL EXAMINATION

Physical examination reveals a normal gait. Discomfort is now minimal. **The patient has localized swelling in the area of the third metatarsal.** The localized swelling indicates a process related to the bone itself. **In addition, this area is tender to palpation, particularly in the area of the third metatarsal neck.** This is a common area for stress fractures, which when healing often produce bony callus. **Lateral compression of the metatarsals is not painful.** Lateral compression usually elicits pain in the case of a Morton's neuroma (interdigital). **Sensory examination is normal.** A neuroma is unlikely.

The fact that the pain is decreasing suggests that the problem is getting better and is most likely to be a healing stress fracture rather than a neoplasm or an inflammation. Morton's neuroma and metatarsalgia are chronic problems more likely to become increasingly painful with time.

LABORATORY FINDINGS
AP and oblique x-rays taken shortly after the onset of pain are presented at left in Fig 7.1. AP and oblique views taken at the time of presentation 2 months later are shown at right in the figure. The later x-rays reveal bony callus formation in the third metatarsal.

HISTORY

The patient is a 26-year-old athletic Peruvian male who presents with right heel pain, which began gradually and has persisted unchanged for 2 months. It is worse upon awakening in the morning and does not increase with activity. He denies any specific injury to the area; however, he is a tennis and racquetball player. Medical history reveals one episode of right elbow tendinitis 1 year ago, which responded to aspirin and ice massage. He has also had intermittent pain around his knees but without redness or swelling. Three months ago he had tendinitis of the extensor pollicis brevis and abductor pollicis longus tendons (de Quervain's disease) and redness in both eyes without any purulent discharge. These resolved after treatment with indomethacin (Indocin). Within the last 2 weeks the patient traveled to Mexico and returned with a mild diarrheal illness and a urethral discharge. The diarrhea has since resolved. The patient's last sexual contacts included one contact with a woman 6 months ago and recently exclusively his current partner. His mother is alive and well; his father died at age 62 of cancer. His father's brother has had painful joints, particularly knees. The patient has three brothers and two sisters, and one of the brothers has painful hands, wrists, and back.

PHYSICAL EXAMINATION

Observation reveals normal lower extremity alignment and no limp. There is no redness or swelling of any joints.

No skin lesions or obvious abnormalities of the iris or the pupil are present. The left conjunctiva is reddened. Palpation of the plantar surface of the calcaneus at the insertion of the plantar fascia produces pain. This pain increases with dorsiflexion of the toes. Ankle and subtalar joint motion is normal, symmetrical, and painless. The chest expansion is 1 inch. Examination of the genitalia reveals a yellow purulent penile discharge but no penile lesions. Rectal examination is normal and stool is guaiac negative.

LABORATORY FINDINGS

Laboratory data include normal CBC, normal ESR, negative ANA, negative RF, and positive HLA-B-27. A lateral x-ray of the heel and ankle area was taken (Fig 7.2).

QUESTIONS

1. In this case, how does one differentiate a mechanical problem from a widespread inflammatory disease process?
2. What is the significance of a 1-inch chest expansion in a patient presenting with foot pain?
3. Explain the possible roles that athletic activity and foreign travel might play in this patient's problem.
4. What additional diagnostic studies should be done at this time?

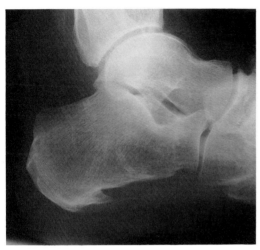

Figure 7.2

Discussion

HISTORY

The patient is a 26-year-old athletic Peruvian male who presents with right heel pain, which began gradually and has persisted unchanged for 2 months. The differential diagnosis of heel pain in a 26-year-old athletic male includes plantar fasciitis, an inflammatory disease, and stress fracture of the calcaneus. **It is worse upon awakening in the morning and does not increase with activity.**

He denies any specific injury to the area; however, he is a tennis and racquetball player. Morning symptoms and the lack of exacerbation with activity suggest an inflammatory disease rather than trauma or a mechanical problem. **Medical history reveals one episode of right elbow tendinitis 1 year ago, which responded to aspirin and ice massage. He has also had intermittent pain around his knees but without redness or swelling. Three months ago he had tendinitis of the extensor pollicis brevis and abductor pollicis longus tendons (de Quervain's disease) and redness in both eyes without any purulent discharge. These resolved after treatment with indomethacin (Indocin).** These suggest a systemic problem that responds to anti-inflammatory medication. A possible diagnosis is Reiter's syndrome, which is a triad of urethritis, arthritis, and iritis or conjunctivitis. All components of the triad need not be present simultaneously. **Within the last 2 weeks, the patient traveled to Mexico and returned with a mild diarrheal illness and a urethral discharge. The diarrhea has since resolved.** Gastrointestinal infection with *Shigella*, *Salmonella*, or *Yersinia* can precipitate Reiter's syndrome in a patient with an HLA-B-27 genotype. Therefore, we might attribute the current problem to his recent diarrheal illness. This patient, however, had a systemic inflammatory illness prior to his trip. **The patient's last sexual contacts included one contact with a woman 6 months ago and recently exclusively his current partner.** Reiter's syndrome may also be due to sexually acquired *Chlamydia* infection. **His mother is alive and well; his father died at age 62 of**

cancer. **His father's brother has had painful joints, particularly knees. The patient has three brothers and two sisters, and one of the brothers has painful hands, wrists, and back.** This history suggests a genetic component to the patient's problem.

PHYSICAL EXAMINATION

Observation reveals normal lower extremity alignment and no limp. There is no redness or swelling of any joints. No synovitis is present. **No skin lesions or obvious abnormalities of the iris or pupil are present. The left conjunctiva is reddened.** The absence of skin lesions does not rule out Reiter's syndrome. When present, skin lesions initially appear as small, red-to-yellowish brown papules, which are nontender. They may then become confluent and hyperkeratotic and be difficult to distinguish from psoriasis when occurring on the palms and soles. Conjunctivitis is present. **Palpation of the plantar surface of the calcaneus at the insertion of the plantar fascia produces pain. This pain increases with dorsiflexion of the toes.** These findings are consistent with plantar fasciitis or os calcis periostitis. One of the common

sites of inflammation in Reiter's syndrome is at entheses (areas where ligaments attach to bone). **Ankle and subtalar joint motion is normal, symmetrical, and painless.** These joints are not currently involved. **The chest expansion is 1 inch.** In a young patient, limited chest expansion (less than 1 inch) reflects early costovertebral joint stiffness. This is often associated with the HLA-B-27 genotype. **Examination of the genitalia reveals a yellow purulent penile discharge but no penile lesions. Rectal examination is normal and stool is guaiac negative.** Urethritis is a component of Reiter's syndrome. The diarrheal illness is not hemorrhagic or currently active.

LABORATORY FINDINGS

Laboratory data include normal CBC, normal ESR, negative ANA, negative RF, and positive HLA-B-27. This patient has no evidence of seropositive rheumatoid arthritis and has the B-27 genotype. **A lateral x-ray of the heel and ankle area was taken (Fig 7.2).** The foot radiograph shows a calcaneal spur resulting from increased plantar fascial tension. Additional diagnostic studies might include stool culture and urethral culture.

Foot Pain

HISTORY

A.K. is a 20-year-old female high-fashion model with a 6-month history of pain on the plantar surfaces of both feet in the area of the metatarsal heads. The pain is particularly aggravated by wearing high-heeled shoes or boots. In her work the patient spends a great deal of time on her feet. Her family history is unremarkable and she has had no other joint problems.

PHYSICAL EXAMINATION

The patient's gait when she is barefooted is normal. Examination of the patient's feet when she is standing reveals no cavus or bunion deformities. The first ray is slightly shorter than the second on both feet, and the configuration of the toes is normal. When the patient is seated, physical examination reveals callosities over the second through the fifth metatarsal heads on both feet, with the largest callosities over the second and third metatarsal heads. These callosities are tender to palpation. The patient cannot dorsiflex either ankle beyond neutral and has 40° plantar flexion bilaterally. Sensation in her toes is normal, and lateral compression of the metatarsal heads is not painful.

QUESTIONS

1. How do you distinguish plantar callosities from plantar warts?
2. What generally produces excessive plantar callosities?
3. Can you relate any of the other physical findings to the presence of the plantar callosities?
4. Why doesn't the first metatarsal head have a callus?
5. How does the effect of shoe wear on the patient's anatomy contribute to metatarsalgia?
6. What other conditions produce metatarsalgia?

Discussion

HISTORY

A.K. is a 20-year-old female high-fashion model with a 6-month history of pain on the plantar surfaces of both feet in the area of the metatarsal heads. The long history essentially rules out any acute injury and makes the problem more likely to be anatomically or occupationally related. Systemic diseases such as rheumatoid arthritis cannot be ruled out. **The pain is particularly aggravated by wearing high-heeled shoes or boots.** This type of shoe forces the patient to put more weight on the metatarsal heads. In addition, the foot is plantarflexed, causing shortening of the Achilles tendons. **In her work the patient spends a great deal of time on her feet.** This history points out that in the course of her work the patient spends a great deal of time loading her metatarsal heads. **Her family history is unremarkable and she has had no other joint problems.** Rheumatoid arthritis, which can produce metatarsalgia, is less likely.

79

PHYSICAL EXAMINATION

The patient's gait when she is barefooted is normal. The absence of a limp is probably a reflection of her decreased activity on the day of the examination. **Examination of the patient's feet when she is standing reveals no cavus or bunion deformities.** A cavus or high-arched foot puts greater force on the metatarsal heads and can contribute to metatarsalgia and callus formation. A bunion can also increase metatarsal head pressure because of lack of support by the first ray. **The first ray is slightly shorter than the second on both feet, and the configuration of the toes is normal.** A foot with a short first ray is called a Morton's foot. Because the first ray is shorter, a greater than normal amount of force is placed on the second metatarsal head, which develops a plantar callus. **When the patient is seated, physical examination reveals callosities over the second through the fifth metatarsal heads on both feet, with the largest callosities over the second and third metatarsal heads. These callosities are tender to palpation.** The finding of callosities predominantly over the second and third metatarsal heads is consistent with the excessive weight borne by these metatarsals in the presence of a short first ray. Plantar warts can be distinguished from callosities because they are often located in areas where there is no mechanical pressure. In addition, if the hyperkeratotic area is gently cut parallel to the surface of the lesion, a callus will be found to have a waxy core whereas a wart will have punctate vascular areas. **The patient cannot dorsiflex either ankle beyond neutral and has 40° plantar flexion bilaterally.** This finding reflects shortened Achilles tendons bilaterally, the result of wearing high-heeled shoes. **Sensation in her toes is normal, and lateral compression of the metatarsal heads is not painful.** When Morton's neuroma is present, lateral compression of the metatarsal heads will produce pain or tingling in the involved toes as the intermetatarsal neuroma is squeezed, and sensation in the involved toes may be abnormal.

HISTORY

R.J. is a 45-year-old male carpenter who presents with right great toe pain of 4 months' duration. The pain developed gradually and is aggravated by walking but is not symptomatic when the patient is not bearing weight. The pain is localized to the metatarsophalangeal joint of the right great toe. More recently the patient has noticed redness and swelling in this area.

PHYSICAL EXAMINATION

Physical examination reveals a healthy male who walks without limping. Inspection of the standing patient reveals diagonal creases across the top of the right shoe, contrasted with horizontal creases across the top of the left shoe (Fig 7.3). Examination of the feet shows no abnormality except for unusually large great toes, which are deviated laterally. The right MTP joint is enlarged, and the soft tissue medially is thickened and red. Palpation medially produces minimal tenderness. Ankle, subtalar, and midfoot motion is normal. Passive great toe range of motion examination reveals the following:

	Right	Left
Dorsiflexion	10°	60°
Plantarflexion	20°	30°
Interphalangeal joint motion	Normal	Normal

LABORATORY FINDINGS

An AP x-ray of the right foot was obtained (Fig 7.4).

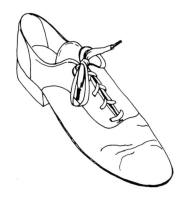

Figure 7.3

QUESTIONS

1. What shoe wear changes are typical of great toe pathology?
2. What anatomic features of his foot predispose to this patient's problem?
3. How do you distinguish the pain in an arthritic metatarsophalangeal joint from that due to an overlying bursitis?

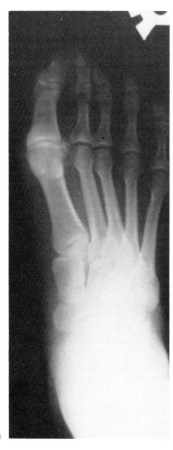

Figure 7.4

Discussion

HISTORY

R.J. is a 45-year-old male carpenter who presents with right great toe pain of 4 months' duration. Pain in a weight-bearing extremity may be caused by a local skin lesion at the point of contact, impact forces on bone and joint, or inflammation of overlying musculotendinous structures. **The pain developed gradually and is aggravated by walking but is not symptomatic when the patient is not bearing weight.** Relief of pain when weight bearing is eliminated suggests bone or joint involvement rather than overlying tendinitis. **The pain is localized to the metatarsophalangeal joint of the right great toe. More recently the patient has noticed redness and swelling in this area.** Redness and swelling are signs of inflammation. Soft-tissue infection would cause pain that would not be relieved by elimination of weight bearing.

PHYSICAL EXAMINATION

Physical examination reveals a healthy male who walks without limping. Either the pain is not severe, or the patient is splinting the MTP joint during the examination. **Inspection of the standing patient reveals diagonal creases across the top of the right shoe, contrasted with horizontal creases across the top of the left shoe (Fig 7.3).** Abnormal wear patterns on the medial side of the sole, abnormal flexion creases, and localized pouching out of the medial side of the shoe upper at the first MTP joint are all characteristic of great toe pathology. The diagonal crease is pathognomonic of diminished motion at the first MTP joint. The crease is diagonal because the axis of motion extends from the tip of the great toe to the MTP joint of the fifth toe. Normally the plane of motion extends transversely across all five MTP joints. **Examination of the feet shows no abnormality except for unusually large great toes, which are deviated laterally.** Since the amount of weight a particular toe bears is proportional to its relative size, these halluces are bearing more weight than the average hallux. Lateral deviation of the great toe is called hallux valgus. **The right MTP joint is enlarged, and the soft tissue medially is thickened and red. Palpation medially produces minimal tenderness.** Enlargement of the MTP joint occurs with degenerative joint disease. Hallux valgus with overlying redness and swelling isolated to the medial side of the MTP joint suggests a bunion. **Ankle, subtalar, and mid-foot motion is normal.** The problem is confined to the MTP joint of the great toe. **Passive great toe range of motion examination reveals the following: (see range of motion chart).** The right MTP joint has a restricted range of motion. First MTP joint enlargement accompanied by restricted MTP joint motion, especially dorsiflexion, is characteristic of degenerative joint disease of the first MTP joint (hallux rigidus). The medial redness and thickening of surrounding soft tissues suggest a bursitis, probably related to the hallux valgus. However, the lack of tenderness suggests that this is not the major problem.

LABORATORY FINDINGS

An AP x-ray of the right foot was obtained (Fig 7.4). The x-ray reveals marked degenerative changes of the first MTP joint. These include loss of the joint space, flattening and sclerosis of the articular surfaces, and spur formation.

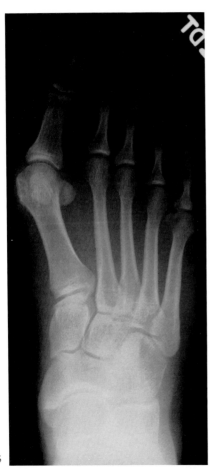

Figure 7.5

HISTORY

A 25-year-old female presents with complaints of right third toe pain of 6 months' duration. The patient works as a salesperson in a department store and must dress fashionably, including the wearing of high-heeled shoes. By the end of the day she experiences severe discomfort between the third and fourth toes. Pain is not present when she is walking barefoot or not bearing weight. She is otherwise in good health, does not smoke, and has never injured that foot.

PHYSICAL EXAMINATION

Examination reveals an attractive woman, fashionably dressed, wearing high-heeled shoes with pointed toes. When standing barefoot the patient displays slight flattening of the medial arch, moderate splaying of her forefoot bilaterally, and at least 15° of hallux valgus. When the patient is sitting, range of motion is normal throughout her foot and ankle. The toes are not deformed. The distribution of callosities over the metatarsal heads is normal. There is no tenderness about the first metatarsophalangeal joint despite the presence of hallux valgus. Some tenderness is present under the third and fourth metatarsal heads. Compressing the right foot from the medial and lateral sides simultaneously causes electric shock-like pains to radiate down into the third and fourth toes. Sensory testing shows some hypesthesia in the third web space. A consistent click is felt when manipulating the third metatarsal with respect to the fourth.

LABORATORY FINDINGS

An AP x-ray of the affected foot was taken (Fig 7.5).

QUESTIONS

1. Describe the deleterious effects that result from wearing high-heeled shoes with pointed toes.
2. How do you distinguish between metatarsalgia and Morton's neuroma (interdigital neuroma)?

Discussion

HISTORY

A 25-year-old female presents with complaints of right third toe pain of 6 months' duration. The toe pain is due to a chronic condition. **The patient works as a salesperson in a department store and must dress fashionably, including the wearing of high-heeled shoes.** High-heeled shoes force the patient to put more weight on her metatarsal heads. Frequent wearing of this type of shoe can lead to toe deformities including hallux valgus and hammer toes. **By the end of the day she experiences severe discomfort between the third and fourth toes.** Pain in the toes can originate from the toes proper, the metatarsal head area, or structures coursing through the web spaces. **Pain is not present when she is walking barefoot or not bearing weight.** Bearing weight in shoes is a component of the problem. Absence of pain when walking barefoot makes metatarsalgia less likely. **She is otherwise in good health, does not smoke, and has never injured that foot.** A nutritional neuropathy, peripheral vascular disease from smoking, and postinjury residua are not present.

PHYSICAL EXAMINATION

Examination reveals an attractive woman, fashionably dressed, wearing high-heeled shoes with pointed toes. In this type of shoe, the toes are driven into the pointed toe box, causing increased friction of the toes against the shoe and squeezing together of the metatarsal heads. **When standing barefoot the patient displays slight flattening of the medial arch, moderate splaying of her forefoot bilaterally, and at least 15° of hallux valgus.** Splaying indicates that her feet spread when bearing weight. Extra-width shoes are usually required to accommodate this type of foot. Flattening of the medial arch when standing results in a valgus force on the great toe. **When the patient is sitting, range of motion is normal throughout her foot and ankle.** Restricted motion is not contributing to the problem. **The toes are not deformed. The distribution of callosities over the metatarsal heads is normal.** Toe deformities, corns, or callosities are not responsible for the pain. **There is no tenderness about the first metatarsophalangeal joint despite the presence of hallux valgus.** The hallux valgus is not causing symptoms. **Some tenderness is present under the third and fourth metatarsal heads.** When metatarsalgia is found in the absence of abnormal callosities, the pain is more likely coming from structures coursing through the webspace.

Compressing the right foot from the medial and lateral sides simultaneously causes electric shock-like pains to radiate down into the third and fourth toes. Paresthesias in these toes suggest impingement of the digital nerve supplying the third web space. Sensory testing shows some hypesthesia in the third web space. Impairment of sensory nerve function is present. A consistent click is felt when manipulating the third metatarsal with respect to the fourth. This finding suggests a soft-tissue lesion between the metatarsal heads, which moves in response to local pressure, and is characteristic of an interdigital (Morton's) neuroma.

LABORATORY FINDINGS

An AP x-ray of the affected foot was taken (Fig 7.5). The x-ray reveals first metatarsal splaying and hallux valgus. This film rules out congenital abnormalities, past trauma, degenerative changes, and other bony lesions as causative factors.

8 Low Back Pain

Low Back Pain (Adult)

Precipitating Event or Cause	Differential Diagnosis	Key Findings	Key Tests	Natural History if Untreated	Treatment	Expected Outcome with Treatment

Trauma
Overuse
  Lifting
  High impact (e.g., tractor)
  Obesity
  Poor posture
Previous surgery
Secondary gain
  Industrial claim
  Litigation
  Justification for dependency
Insidious (no overt event)
	Sprain/strain	Activity-related	None	Intermittent pain	Exercises
					NSAID
						Recurrence

	Herniated disk	Nerve root tension signs	EMG Myelogram CT	Gradual resolution	Bed rest	Recurrence
				Progressive deficit	Laminectomy	
	Fracture	Local percussion tenderness	X-ray CT	Healing	Support (internal or external)	Intermittent pain
	Tumor	Persistence with night pain	Bone scan CT MRI	Destruction	Chemotherapy Radiation Surgery	Pain relief if structural integrity preserved Deformity if structural deficiency Depends on tumor type

NSAID, Nonsteroidal anti-inflammatory drug; EMG, electromyography; CT, computed tomography; MRI, magnetic resonance imaging.

Precipitating Event or Cause	Differential Diagnosis	Key Findings	Key Tests	Natural History if Untreated	Treatment	Expected Outcome with Treatment
Trauma Overuse Lifting	Spinal stenosis	Leg pain when walking, relieved by sitting	Myelogram CT scan MRI	Intermittent pain Reduced ambulatory tolerance	Spinal canal decompression	Ambulation restored Intermittent back pain

High impact (e.g., tractor)
Obesity
Poor posture
Previous surgery
Secondary gain
  Industrial claim
  Litigation
  Justification for dependency
Insidious (no overt event)
	Spondyloarthropathy (e.g., ankylosing spondylitis, psoriasis, enteropathies)	Decreased chest expansion	Positive HLA-B-27	Decreased range of motion
				Deformity
					Postural exercise
					NSAID
						Decreased range of motion
						Minimize or prevent deformity

	Vertebral osteomyelitis	Local percussion tenderness	Needle biopsy Culture	Gradual destruction Autofusion	Antibiotics Immobilization	Autofusion
	Spondylolisthesis	Tight hamstrings Increased lordosis	Vertebral slip on lateral x-ray Pars defect on oblique x-rays	Not always symptomatic No further slippage if over 20 years of age	Brace Postural exercise Fusion	May or may not be symptomatic
	Chronic pain syndrome	Pain behavior Secondary gain	MMPI	Persistence	Multidisciplinary	Major improvement unlikely

CT, computed tomography; MRI, magnetic resonance imaging; MMPI, Minnesota Multiphasic Personality Inventory; NSAID, nonsteroidal anti-inflammatory drugs.

HISTORY

This 29-year-old white male office worker presents with a 6-week history of low back pain radiating down the anterior aspect of the left thigh and left leg. The onset was acute, occurring with a hard sneeze. There was no antecedent trauma. The leg pain increases with activity, Valsalva maneuvers, and extension of the leg. It decreases with flexion of the waist. There has been no numbness, weakness, or change in bowel or bladder habits. The patient has not improved after a period of 6 weeks of strict bed rest.

PHYSICAL EXAMINATION

On physical examination the patient lists forward and to the right. Heel and toe walking are normal. On forward flexion the fingertips fail to reach the floor by 24 inches. He returns to the upright position with marked dysrhythmia. The patient cannot extend his lumbar spine because of spasms. Tests of motor strength show grade 4 quadriceps on the left. The remainder of the motor examination is normal. Sensation is intact. Deep tendon reflexes are left knee 1+, right knee 2+, both ankle jerks 2+. Babinski's sign is absent. The straight leg raising test is positive at 30°, with pain radiating down the left lower extremity. The cross straight leg raising test is negative. The reverse straight leg raising test is markedly positive on the left. Past medical history is unremarkable.

QUESTIONS

1. What is the significance of pain radiating down an extremity?
2. What are the important signs of progressing neurologic impairment?
3. What is the significance of an increase in pain with Valsalva maneuvers (cough, sneeze, laugh, strain)?
4. How are the following used in assessment of the patient with back pain?
   A. Listing
   B. Tension signs
   C. Dynamic alignment
5. Explain why forward flexion relieves the pain whereas extension increases it.
6. What back conditions can be excluded?
7. What additional workup is required to do so?
8. At what level does the problem exist?

Discussion

HISTORY

This 29-year-old white male office worker presents with a 6-week history of low back pain radiating down the anterior aspect of the left thigh and left leg. Pain radiating down an extremity suggests nerve root irritation. However, nonradiating, aching pain in the leg may be referred from facet joints, a bulging annulus, or other nonneural structures in the back. Referred pain is pain present at a site distant from the site of origin of the pain but related in sclerotomal development to that site. **The onset was acute, occurring with a hard sneeze. There was no antecedent trauma.** This tends to eliminate fracture and muscle strain as diagnoses. An acute disk herniation may occur without obvious cause. **The leg pain increases with activity, Valsalva maneuvers, and extension of the leg.** These are all tension signs indicative of nerve root irritation. **It decreases with flexion of the waist.** Flexion of the lumbar spine opens the foramina, providing more space for the nerve roots. **There has been no numbness, weakness, or change in bowel or bladder habits.** Major neurologic deficit is unlikely, nor has the neurologic impairment progressed. **The patient has not improved after a period of 6 weeks of strict bed rest.** Ninety percent of patients with low back pain have recovered by 6 weeks.

PHYSICAL EXAMINATION

On physical examination the patient lists forward and to the right. He is adopting a posture that relieves nerve root tension. A list is an obligatory posture produced by secondary muscle spasm in response to nerve root tension. **Heel and toe walking are normal.** This indicates that lower extremity muscle strength is essentially normal and symmetrical. **On forward flexion the fingertips fail to reach the floor by 24 inches. He returns to the upright position with marked dysrhythmia. The patient cannot extend his lumbar spine because of spasms.** This dysrhythmia and the limitation of movement in the lumbar spine indicate muscle splinting. **Tests of motor strength show grade 4 quadriceps on the left. The remainder of the motor examination is normal. Sensation is intact. Deep tendon reflexes are left knee 1+, right knee 2+, both ankle jerks 2+.** There is minimal involvement of the L-3 or L-4 nerve supply to the left quadriceps muscle. The decreased left knee jerk also reflects L-3 or L-4 nerve root irritation. **Babinski's sign is absent.** No upper motor neuron lesion is present. **The straight leg raising test is positive at 30°, with pain radiating down the left lower extremity.** The nerve roots begin to move in the foramina at 25° to 30° of straight leg raising. **The cross straight leg raising test is negative.** A positive cross straight leg raising test is present if pain radiates down the symptomatic leg when the opposite leg is raised. This is strongly suggestive of nerve root impingement. **The reverse straight leg raising test is markedly positive on the left.** The reverse straight leg raising test is performed with the patient prone and stretches the femoral nerve and its roots (L-2 through L-4). The positive test indicates impingement of one or more of these roots. **Past medical history is unremarkable.** This tends to make systemic causes of low back pain (such as infection or tumor) less likely.

Additional workup should include myelogram or CT scan to identify the problem and its anatomic level (most likely the L3–4 interspace).

HISTORY

This 38-year-old white male veteran is seen because of chronic low back pain of 14 months' duration. The pain began suddenly when he caught a falling 100-lb object while his back was partially bent. This incident occurred while on active duty in the armed forces. A subsequent evaluation at a nearby naval hospital included a myelogram. The overall picture seemed to warrant exploration, and the patient underwent an L-5, S-1 discectomy. No herniated disk was found. On the third day postoperatively the patient experienced severe left leg pain and numbness. He later developed pain and numbness down the right leg. These symptoms have persisted for the past 13 months and are incapacitating. Occasionally he can produce a "popping" in his back, following which the left leg is "completely dead." He is unable to lie on a soft surface and usually sits with difficulty propped on his left buttock. Ambulation aggravates the leg pain. Valsalva maneuvers do not. Bed rest does not improve the pain. Bowel and bladder habits have not changed. Treatment has consisted of various anti-inflammatory medications, analgesics including Tylenol 3, and three to six beers per day.

PHYSICAL EXAMINATION

Physical examination shows a well-developed male sitting uncomfortably perched on his right buttock and supporting himself with both arms. Examination of the back reveals a well-healed midline lower lumbar scar.

When standing, the patient has a normal lumbar lordosis with no pelvic tilt or paraspinous muscle spasm. When he bends forward from a standing position, his fingertips fail to reach the floor by 2½ feet, and the lumbar lordosis reverses. The patient walks with an antalgic gait favoring the left leg. He can heel and toe walk but favors the left leg. There is tenderness overlying the scar. Motor examination shows grade IV (out of V) muscle strength in both lower extremities. However, during strength testing the left lower extremity moves in a jerking, cogwheel fashion. In the left lower extremity sensation of pinprick is without dermatomal distribution and is diffusely duller than in the right. Reflexes are 2+ and symmetrical at the knee and the ankle. Babinski's sign is absent. Left straight leg raising to 10° produces diffuse left lower extremity pain; right straight leg raising to 70° produces diffuse right lower extremity pain.

LABORATORY FINDINGS

X-rays (not shown) reveal a normal lumbar spine. An electromyogram reveals membrane instability in the L-5, S-1 right paraspinal muscles. An MMPI (Minnesota Multiphasic Personality Inventory) shows a conversion V pattern. Consulting psychologists feel the patient has a mild thought disorder held in check by somatization and denial.

QUESTIONS

1. To what extent is the history supported by the physical findings?

2. What are the red flags in this case?
3. How does one distinguish between functional and organic pathology in the patient presenting with low back pain?

Discussion

HISTORY

This 38-year-old white male veteran is seen because of chronic low back pain of 14 months' duration. The pain began suddenly when he caught a falling 100-lb object while his back was partially bent. The mechanism of injury is significant in that doing any heavy lifting with the back bent forward exerts great force on the lumbar spine. Catching a heavy falling object would increase this force. **This incident occurred while on active duty in the armed forces.** As a veteran the patient is "service-connected" for this injury and may be eligible for disability pay. A review board must weigh the facts and opinions in the case and decide on the nature and extent of the disability. **A subsequent evaluation at a nearby naval hospital included a myelogram. The overall picture seemed to warrant exploration, and the patient underwent an L-5, S-1 discectomy. No herniated disk was found.** The results of the evaluation and the myelogram are not known. However, we must assume that the findings were sufficiently positive to warrant disk exploration. In general, a progressive neurologic deficit and a related filling defect on myelogram warrant exploration.

A negative disk exploration indicates an error of patient selection for surgery or failure to locate the abnormal disk. Removing a normal disk may cause future back problems. **On the third day postoperatively the patient experienced severe left leg pain and numbness. He later developed pain and numbness down the right leg.** These symptoms could be caused by surgical nerve root irritation or extravasation of disk material that was not removed at the time of surgery. **These symptoms have persisted for the past 13 months and are incapacitating.** Most individuals who develop back pain from either mechanical causes or nerve root impingement from a herniated disk experience relief in 3 to 4 months from bed rest and activity precautions. We do not know how this patient was treated. That these symptoms have persisted for 13 months and are "incapacitating" is inconsistent with the usual natural history of mechanical or acute disk problems. **Occasionally he can produce a "popping" in his back, following which the left leg is "completely dead."** This kind of exotic history is highly suspicious and without anatomic basis. **He is unable to lie on a soft surface and usually sits with difficulty propped on his left buttock.** Soft surfaces do not support the spine and tend to aggravate low back pain. Sitting propped up on the left buttock may change the alignment of the lumbar spine in a way that relieves pain. **Ambulation aggravates the leg pain.** Walking requires some movement of the lumbar spine, which can aggravate nerve roots already under tension. **Valsalva maneuvers do not.** Valsalva maneuvers raise intradural pressure and produce more ten-

93

sion on the nerve roots. One would expect pain from an acute radiculopathy to be aggravated by Valsalva maneuvers. **Bed rest does not improve the pain.** Spine tumors can cause night and rest pain. Spine x-rays and bone scans are helpful in diagnosing tumors. **Bowel and bladder habits have not changed.** Cauda equina impingement is unlikely. **Treatment has consisted of various anti-inflammatory medications, analgesics, including Tylenol 3, and three to six beers per day.** Anti-inflammatory medications are indicated for degenerative joint disease of the lumbar spine, a condition unlikely in this 38-year-old male. Consumption of alcohol for pain control requires further investigation into the patient's social history.

PHYSICAL EXAMINATION

Physical examination shows a well-developed male sitting uncomfortably perched on his right buttock and supporting himself with both arms. This is inconsistent with the patient's statement that he has to sit propped up on his left buttock. **Examination of the back reveals a well-healed midline lower lumbar scar.** The patient has undergone back surgery. **When standing, the patient has a normal lumbar lordosis with no pelvic tilt or paraspinous muscle spasm.** Acute disc herniations are usually associated with listing and a loss of lumbar lordosis. **When he bends forward from a standing position, his fingertips fail to reach the floor by 2½ feet, and the lumbar lordosis reverses.** This limited motion can result from lumbar muscle spasm, hamstring tightness, low back discomfort,

or lack of patient cooperation. Complete reversal of the lumbar lordosis on forward flexion means spasm is not present. **The patient walks with an antalgic gait favoring the left leg.** The patient's left leg or back hurts during stance phase on the left leg. Watching the patient walk and undress reveals the degree of functional disability. **The patient can heel and toe walk but favors the left leg.** This is a dynamic motor function test of the plantar and dorsiflexors of the foot. The test is normal in this patient. **There is tenderness overlying the scar.** This is a suspicious finding in that most scars eventually become insensitive. **Motor examination shows grade IV (out of V) muscle strength in both lower extremities.** This level of muscle strength means that there is a perceptible but minimal decrease in motor strength compared to normal. This subjective test is not consistent with the normal heel and toe walking noted above. **However, during strength testing the left lower extremity moves in a jerking, cogwheel fashion.** This is an inappropriate response to strength testing. The weakness may be more functional than organic. **In the left lower extremity, sensation of pinprick is without dermatomal distribution and is diffusely duller than in the right.** This picture is not consistent with a specific nerve root pattern. **Reflexes are 2+ and symmetrical at the knee and the ankle. Babinski's sign is absent.** An upper motor neuron lesion is unlikely. **Left straight leg raising to 10° produces diffuse left lower extremity pain; right straight leg raising to 70° produces diffuse right lower extremity pain.** Ipsilateral and contralateral straight leg raising may increase sciatic nerve root tension on the involved side. The contralateral straight leg raising sign (cross straight leg raising sign) is positive when elevating the contralateral leg reproduces the patient's sciatica. When nerve root entrapment is present, sciatic tension causes pain to radiate down the leg. The leg must be raised to at least 30° before significant sciatic tension is produced. Straight leg raising beyond 40° causes minimal additional tension. The findings in this patient do not indicate nerve root entrapment.

LABORATORY FINDINGS

X-rays reveal a normal lumbar spine. An electromyogram reveals membrane instability in the L5, S1 right paraspinal muscles. This is a common, nonspecific finding in patients with low back pain. **An MMPI** (Minnesota Multiphasic Personality Inventory) **shows a conversion V pattern.** The MMPI was originally developed to assess disabling psychological abnormalities. The test consists of 550 items, which separate into ten clinical psychological scales and three validity scales. In low back pain the most important indication of somatic fixation has been the conversion V of the neurotic triad. The conversion V pattern consists of an abnormal elevation of hypochondriasis (scale 1) and hysteria (scale 3) above depression (scale 2). Individuals demonstrating a conversion V pattern complain of physical symptoms but display indifference or apparent dissociation of affective reactions. The test is used by the surgeon to help sort out whether the patient's back pain is organic or primarily functional. Other factors that suggest functional pain include inconsistent physical findings, "pain behavior" (exaggerated responses), and secondary gain. Organic problems usually produce symptoms consistent with an anatomic lesion. **Consulting psychologists feel the patient has a mild thought disorder held in check by somatization and denial.** This is one of the many interpretations of a conversion V pattern.

HISTORY

This 60-year-old male presents with a 2-month history of low back pain. The pain began several days following a minor twisting injury to the knee, which caused the patient to limp. The pain grew increasingly worse until it became constant and awakened the patient at night. For the past 2 weeks, the patient has been on complete bed rest at home and unable to continue his job as an office worker. Although somewhat better on bed rest, the pain is still increased by ambulation. The pain radiates down the front of the left leg to the left knee. The patient has noted no numbness or weakness. He has urinary incontinence following a radical prostatectomy 2 years ago for carcinoma of the prostate.

PHYSICAL EXAMINATION

The patient appears somewhat ill and in moderate distress when asked to move about and walk. In the standing position he shows no scoliosis or list. Percussion of the spinous processes reveals diffuse tenderness throughout the lower lumbar area. Forward bend is smooth and symmetrical, with the fingertips failing to reach the floor by 1½ feet. There is no jerking or muscle spasm on returning to the upright position. Sensory and motor examination reveals no abnormalities. In the sitting position the patient's knee and ankle reflexes are 2+ and symmetrical. Babinski's sign is not present. Supine, the patient demonstrates full range of motion of his hips. Straight leg raising and Patrick's tests are negative.

LABORATORY FINDINGS

Liver scan, chest x-rays (not shown), and barium enema 4 months ago revealed no metastases. Hematocrit is 41, ESR 54, white blood cell count 9,100, alkaline phosphatase 720, and SGOT (serum glutamic oxaloacetic transaminase) 10.

QUESTIONS

1. How does the clinical picture in this patient differ from that in the patient with strained back muscles?
2. What further laboratory studies might be useful in making a diagnosis?

Discussion

HISTORY

This 60-year-old male presents with a 2-month history of low back pain. Most low back pain due to minor muscle strains has disappeared by this time. **The pain began several days following a minor twisting injury to the knee, which caused the patient to limp.** Abnormal gait and posture over a period of time may cause low back pain. **The pain grew increasingly worse until it became constant and awakened the patient at night.** Pain due to mechanical causes is lessened by rest and recumbency. Night pain is associated with infection or malignancy. **For the past 2 weeks, the patient has been on complete bed rest at home and unable to continue his job as an office worker. Although somewhat better on bed rest, the pain is still increased by ambulation.** Complete bed rest on a firm mattress ensures that the back has adequate support and is not subject to the shear and compressive forces created by activities of daily living. **The pain radiates down the front of the leg to the left knee.** Radiating pain is indicative of nerve root irritation. This distribution indicates L-3 or L-4 root irritation. **The patient has noted no numbness or weakness.** Significant nerve root impingement or progressive neurologic disorder is unlikely. **He has urinary incontinence following a radical prostatectomy 2 years ago for carcinoma of the prostate.** Knowledge of the patient's prostatic cancer, the tendency for carcinoma of the prostate to metastasize to the spine, and the presence of night pain together strongly suggest that this patient's low back pain is caused by metastatic prostate cancer.

PHYSICAL EXAMINATION

The patient appears somewhat ill and in moderate distress when asked to move about and walk. The impact of the illness on the patient's musculoskeletal system can be assessed by watching the patient stand, walk, and undress. **In the standing position he shows no scoliosis or list.** A list is an objective finding indicating muscle spasm usually due to nerve root irritation. Scoliosis can be primary and structural or secondary to muscle spasm or leg length inequality. **Percussion of the spinous processes reveals diffuse tenderness throughout the lower lumbar area.** Diffuse tenderness is more consistent with a systemic process, whereas local tenderness can be associated with strain, degenerative disk disease, infection, or fracture. **Forward bend is smooth and symmetrical,** with the fingertips failing to reach the floor by 1½ feet. **There is no jerking or muscle spasm on returning to the upright position.** The smooth and symmetrical forward bend is inconsistent with muscle spasm. **Sensory and motor examination reveals no abnormalities. In the sitting position the patient's knee and ankle reflexes are 2+ and symmetrical.** There is no neurologic deficit. **Babinski's sign is not present.** An upper motor neuron lesion is not present. **Supine, the patient demonstrates full range of motion of his hips.** The source of the patient's pain is not in his hips. **Straight leg raising and Patrick's tests are negative.** Straight leg raising produces tension on the sciatic nerve. When lower lumbar nerve root entrapment is present, radiating pain down the ipsilateral leg will occur. Dorsiflexion of the ankle at this point will aggravate symptoms. Patrick's test is used to detect sacroiliac joint pain. The spondyloarthropathies are frequently associated with sacroiliitis.

LABORATORY FINDINGS

Liver scan, chest x-rays (not shown), and barium enema 4 months ago revealed no metastases. This information does not rule out metastases at present. **Hematocrit is 41, ESR 54, white blood cell count 9,100, alkaline phosphatase 720, and SGOT (serum glutamic oxaloacetic transaminase) 10.** The ESR is abnormal, as is the alkaline phosphatase. The clinical picture and the elevated alkaline phosphatase are consistent with metastatic disease involving bone. Bone scan, CT, myelography, and serum acid phosphatase would be useful in confirming the diagnosis.

Low Back Pain

HISTORY

B.B. is a 16-year-old gymnast with low back pain. She has been active in gymnastics for 8 years but has had pain only recently. The pain began insidiously 3 months ago, resolved, and then returned at greater intensity so that the patient was unable to compete. The patient is usually quite competitive and has been practicing year-round both in high school and with a gymnastics club. The pain is localized in her lower back and is present only during gymnastic activities. It is aggravated by maneuvers that hyperextend the spine. The patient has had no radiation of pain into her legs. She feels that she has lost flexibility, because previously she could touch her palms to the floor on forward bending, whereas now she can barely reach the floor with her fingertips. Her history is also positive for intermittent wrist pain while competing. This has resolved since she has been resting. Her history is otherwise unremarkable.

PHYSICAL EXAMINATION

Physical examination reveals a healthy teenage girl with hyperlordotic posture. Her gait is normal. The patient is able to reach forward and touch the floor with her fingertips. Hyperextension and lateral bending are normal and painless. There is no paravertebral spasm or dysrhythmia. There is no tenderness to palpation of her back and no difference in prominence of the lumbar spinous processes. Her neurological examination is entirely normal. Deep tendon reflexes are 2+ at the ankles and 1+ at the knees. Straight leg raising is negative to 100°.

QUESTIONS

1. In what ways might intensive gymnastics cause back problems?
2. When doing a straight leg raising test, how do you distinguish nerve root irritation from hamstring tightness?
3. What further diagnostic studies would be useful?

Discussion

HISTORY

B.B. is a 16-year-old gymnast with low back pain. Many gymnastic maneuvers involve hyperextending the lumbar spine. **She has been active in gymnastics for 8 years but has had pain only recently. The pain began insidiously 3 months ago, resolved, and then returned at greater intensity so that the patient was unable to compete.** The insidious onset is consistent with a low-grade infection, a tumor, or a mild type of overuse problem such as a strain or a stress fracture. **The patient is usually quite competitive and has been practicing year-round both in high school and with a gymnastics club.** This patient spends many hours a week practicing and would be subject to overuse problems. **The pain is localized in her lower back and is present only during gymnastic activities.** These activities make her problem symptomatic. Pain from infection and tumor is present constantly and is not affected by activity. **It is aggravated by maneuvers that hyperextend the spine.** Hyperextending the spine increases stress on the posterior elements of the spine. **The patient has had no radiation of pain into her legs. She feels that she has lost flexibility, because previously she could touch her palms to the floor on forward bending, whereas now she can barely reach the floor with her fingertips.** Inability to touch the floor with the fingertips can be caused by problems in the back or hip or by hamstring tightness. Hamstring spasm is a common concomitant of spondylolysis and spondylolisthesis. **Her history is also positive for intermittent wrist pain while competing. This has resolved since she has been resting.** Gymnasts frequently get capsulitis in the wrist from using the arms as weight-bearing extremities. **Her history is otherwise unremarkable.**

PHYSICAL EXAMINATION

Physical examination reveals a healthy teenage girl with hyperlordotic posture. Hyperlordosis is common in gymnasts. It may arise from chronic hyperlordotic positioning, which also increases hamstring tension. **Her gait is normal.** There is no evidence of spasticity or weakness. **The patient is able to reach forward and touch the floor with her fingertips.** Although this range of motion might be excellent in the normal population, it suggests decreased back or hip range of motion and/or hamstring tightness

in this patient, who is ordinarily able to put her palms on the floor. **Hyperextension and lateral bending are normal and painless. There is no paravertebral spasm or dysrhythmia.** Spasm and dysrhythmia are objective signs that reflect a patient's involuntary attempt to splint an acutely painful back. This patient's condition is not acutely painful. **There is no tenderness to palpation of her back and no difference in prominence of the lumbar spinous processes.** With an acute spondylolysis palpation of the spinous processes produces pain. If a spondylolisthesis (forward slipping of a vertebra) has occurred, one can often palpate a step-off between the lumbar spinous processes. **Her neurological examination is entirely normal. Deep tendon reflexes are 2+ at the ankles and 1+ at the knees.** There is no evidence of serious nerve root impingement. **Straight leg raising is negative to 100°.** Straight leg raising is a test for nerve root irritation. When nerve root irritation is present, pressure in the popliteal fossa or dorsiflexion of the foot will exacerbate the pain. Hamstring tightness alone produces limited motion but no associated pain during the straight leg raising test. A gymnast should be able to perform straight leg raising beyond 100°. A bone scan would distinguish an acute pars interarticularis stress fracture from a long-standing spondylolysis.

9 Shoulder Pain

Shoulder Pain

Precipitating Event or Cause	Differential Diagnosis	Key Findings	Key Tests	Natural History if Untreated	Treatment	Expected Outcome with Treatment
Trauma (direct or indirect) Overuse (especially overhead reach) Insidious (no precipitating event) Metabolic disease Visceral disease	Rotator cuff tear	Weak external rotation Supraspinatus atrophy Painful arc 60°–120° Difficulty initiating abduction	Subacromial dye extravasation on arthrogram	Small tear: Symptoms resolve No functional disability	Cuff-strengthening exercises	Slightly decreased strength in external rotation and abduction
				Large tear: Persistent weakness Atrophy, pain	Repair	Slightly decreased range of motion Slightly decreased strength
				Impingement	Surgery	Resolution
	Supraspinatus tendinitis	Point tenderness Pain with external rotation	Calcification on x-ray	Resolution or recurrence	NSAID	Resolution Possible recurrence
				Impingement	Acromioplasty	Resolution
	Biceps tendinitis	Positive Yergason's test Tender bicipital groove	None	Resolution	NSAID Restrict activity	Slightly decreased supination strength
				Rupture if condition persists	Surgery (biceps stapling)	Resolution
	Impingement syndrome	Acromial pain on humeral forward flexion beyond 90° (Symptoms of cuff tear, tendinitis, bursitis)	Reduced pain with subacromial lidocaine	Resolution	NSAID Subacromial steroid injection (× 3 max.) Cuff-strengthening exercises	Resolution Possible recurrence
				Persistence beyond 9 months	Acromioplasty	Resolution

NSAID, nonsteroidal anti-inflammatory drugs.

Precipitating Event or Cause	Differential Diagnosis	Key Findings	Key Tests	Natural History if Untreated	Treatment	Expected Outcome with Treatment
Trauma (direct or indirect) Overuse (especially overhead reach) Insidious (no precipitating event) Metabolic disease Visceral disease	Frozen shoulder	Decreased passive glenohumeral motion	Reduced capsular space on arthrogram	60% resolve in 2 years If traumatic: persistence	Range-of-motion exercises	Slightly decreased range of motion
	Glenohumeral arthritis	Increased pain with activity Barometric sensitivity	X-ray	Intermittent pain	NSAID	Intermittent activity-related pain
				Progressive	Arthroplasty	Pain relief
	AC joint arthritis	AC joint tenderness and pain with adduction	X-ray Decrease in pain with AC joint lidocaine	Intermittent pain	NSAID AC joint steroid injection (× 3 max.)	Pain relief of variable duration
				Progressive	Distal clavicle resection	Normal function
	Humeral head fracture	History of trauma Local tenderness	X-ray	Healing	Support (internal or external)	Decreased range of motion
	Cervical nerve root impingement	Radicular pain Normal shoulder examination	C-spine x-ray EMG	Intermittent flares Slow to resolve	NSAID Cervical collar Traction Fusion if refractory	Intermittent pain
	Referred pain	Visceral disease (heart or gallbladder)	Related to visceral diagnosis	Resolution	Treat visceral disease	Resolution of shoulder pain
		Normal neck and shoulder exam		Possible frozen shoulder or shoulder-hand syndrome	(See frozen shoulder) Sympathetic blocks Physical therapy	(See frozen shoulder)

NSAID, nonsteroidal anti-inflammatory drugs; AC, acromioclavicular; EMG, electromyography.

HISTORY

A 45-year-old male office worker presents with right shoulder pain and weakness of 24 hours' duration. The patient was skiing down steep terrain when his skis crossed, throwing him forcibly into a nearby mogul. Most of the impact was taken by the right shoulder. Excruciating pain was followed by inability to move the shoulder actively in a normal fashion. Since medical attention was not available, the ski patrol placed the patient's right arm in a sling, and he has come to you for evaluation and further management.

PHYSICAL EXAMINATION

On physical examination the patient is wearing a sling on his right arm and appears mildly uncomfortable. After careful removal of the sling, inspection of the right shoulder reveals swelling anteriorly but no ecchymosis or deformity. Generalized tenderness to palpation is present anteriorly. The patient is unable to actively abduct or forward flex the right shoulder but can reach his right hip pocket. All attempted shoulder movement is painful. Passive range of motion is full, but crepitation is felt anteriorly during forward flexion. External rotation strength is 5+/5 on the left and 3+/5 on the right.

LABORATORY FINDINGS

X-rays of the shoulder (not shown) include AP views of the glenohumeral joint with the humerus internally and externally rotated and an axillary view. No evidence of acromioclavicular joint separation, glenohumeral subluxation/dislocation, or fracture is present.

QUESTIONS

1. What injuries might you expect from a fall directly on the shoulder?
2. How does the patient's age affect the type of injury you expect?
3. How do you distinguish between weakness caused by:
   A. Pain inhibition?
   B. Neurologic deficit?
   C. Skeletal and soft-tissue deficiencies?

Discussion

HISTORY

A 45-year-old male office worker presents with right shoulder pain and weakness of 24 hours' duration. Patients in this age group may sustain degenerative tears of tendons or ligaments. **The patient was skiing down steep terrain when his skis crossed, throwing him forcibly into a nearby mogul.** The cause of the right shoulder problem is trauma. Weakness could be due to pain, direct damage to shoulder structures, or traction injury of the brachial plexus. One should suspect a rotator cuff injury in a male of this age since degenerative changes make the cuff more susceptible to injury. **Most of the impact was taken by the right shoulder.** A significant traumatic event took place. Falls directly on the shoulder can produce contusions; fractures of the humerus, clavicle, or acromion; separation of the acromioclavicular joint, rotator cuff tears, or brachial plexus injuries. **Excruciating pain was followed by inability to move the shoulder actively in a normal fashion.** Given this injury mechanism, this picture could be caused by brachial plexus or suprascapular nerve injury, rotator cuff injury, or humeral fracture. **Since medical attention was not available, the ski patrol placed the patient's right arm in a sling, and he has come to you for further evaluation and management.** The ski patrol performed standard first aid treatment for an upper extremity injury of this type.

PHYSICAL EXAMINATION

On physical exaination the patient is wearing a sling on his right arm and appears mildly uncomfortable. After careful removal of the sling, inspection of the right shoulder reveals swelling anteriorly but no ecchymosis or deformity. Swelling suggests a response to direct contusion. Absence of ecchymosis and deformity is not consistent with a fracture. **Generalized tenderness to palpation is present anteriorly.** This is consistent with a severe contusion. **The patient is unable to actively abduct or forward flex the right shoulder but can reach his right hip pocket.** This finding would suggest incompetence of the rotator cuff due to either neurologic injury, structural deficiency, or pain inhibition. Neurologic injury will be detectible by EMG after 10 days from the time of injury. Atrophy will eventually occur. Skeletal

structural deficiency is demonstrated on x-ray, and soft-tissue tears on arthrography. Pain inhibition can be diagnosed if full shoulder function returns after subacromial lidocaine injection. The rotator cuff muscles stabilize the humeral head during abduction and forward flexion and also are partly responsible for active abduction. Incompetence of the rotator cuff may also produce a shrugging motion on attempted abduction as the unconstrained humeral head rides cephalad. **All attempted shoulder movement is painful.** This finding can represent severe contusion even in the absence of soft-tissue disruption or fracture. The injury seems limited to the shoulder and is unlikely to involve neighboring neural structures. **Passive range of motion is full, but crepitation is felt anteriorly during forward flexion.** Skeletal integrity is intact. Crepitation felt anteriorly is due to soft-tissue impingement underneath the acromial arch. This may be caused by rotator cuff disruption or, in the nontraumatic setting, by bursitis and calcific tendinitis. **External rotation strength is 5+/5 on the left and 3+/5 on the right.** External rotation strength is decreased on the right. This further corroborates the suspicion of rotator cuff tear.

LABORATORY FINDINGS

X-rays of the shoulder (not shown) include AP views of the glenohumeral joint, with the humerus internally and externally rotated, and an axillary view. No evidence of acromioclavicular joint separation, glenohumeral subluxation/dislocation, or fracture is present. Bony structures are intact.

HISTORY

A 35-year-old right-handed housewife and part-time university student in psychology presents with neck and right shoulder pain of 3 weeks' duration. She was driving home from class when another car ran a red light and struck her car on the left front fender. She was wearing a seat belt, had some prior warning that the accident was going to occur, and braced herself but was still thrown violently against the seat belt. Her sunglasses flew off her head. Estimated impact velocity was about 35 mph. Extensive damage was done to the front end and the left front fender. The patient was able to get out of the car and take information from witnesses, but by the next morning she had developed severe midline neck pain and an inability to move her right shoulder without discomfort. Over the next 5 days the neck and right shoulder pain gradually began to subside. By the 14th day the patient had recovered to the extent that she was able to return to her studies. However, over the succeeding week she developed increasing neck and right shoulder discomfort.

PHYSICAL EXAMINATION

Physical examination reveals a well-developed, slightly obese female who walks without a limp. She demonstrates limited forward flexion and incomplete extension of the cervical spine. There is decreased motion on right lateral rotation. Cervical range of motion is otherwise full. The upper extremities demonstrate normal contours and no atrophy. There is point tenderness along the right anterior acromial border. Passive range of motion of the right shoulder is comfortable except on foward flexion beyond 90°, when there is pain in the acromial region. Upper extremity motor and sensory tests reveal no deficits. Supination of the forearm against resistance (Yergason's test for bicipital tendinitis) is painless.

LABORATORY FINDINGS

Radiographs of the cervical spine (not shown) are normal. Fig 9.1 shows AP radiographs of the patient's right shoulder in external (left) and internal (right) rotation views.

QUESTIONS

1. Describe the mechanism of injury and its relationship to the findings.
2. How do you explain the lack of pain initially followed by severe pain later?
3. What injuries to the neck and shoulder might occur with this type of accident, and how would they be ruled out?
4. What is the relationship between the shoulder and the neck pain?

Discussion

HISTORY

A 35-year-old right-handed housewife and part-time university student in psychology presents with neck and right shoulder pain of 3 weeks' duration. Neck and

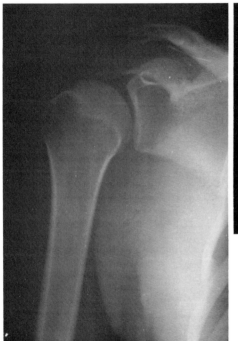 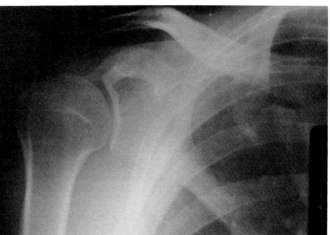

Figure 9.1

shoulder pain frequently occur together and may be related or unrelated. One must distinguish local from radicular or referred pain. **She was driving home from class when another car ran a red light and struck her car on the left front fender.** This mechanism of injury would produce a sudden stop, with the driver being thrown forward and then backward. Both anterior and posterior neck muscles may be stretched or torn by this mechanism. **She was wearing a seat belt, had some prior warning that the accident was going to occur, and braced herself but was still thrown violently against the seat belt. Her sunglasses flew off her head.** This description suggests a high rate of deceleration. **Estimated impact velocity was 35 mph. Extensive damage was done to the front end and the left front fender.** This confirms a high energy of impact. **The patient was able to get out of the car and take information from witnesses, but by the next morning she had developed severe midline neck pain and an inability to move her right shoulder without discomfort.** The severity of injury can be assessed by the rapidity with which symptoms develop. Fractures and dislocations are usually painful immediately, whereas muscle strains may not become painful until 24 hours after injury. Advance warning and wearing restraints mitigated the effects of the impact. **Over the next 5 days the neck and right shoulder pain gradually began to subside. By the 14th day the patient had recovered to the extent that she was able to return to her studies.** Minor neck sprains sustained in automobile accidents usually subside over 1 to 3 weeks. **However, over the succeeding week she developed increasing neck and right shoulder discomfort.** Recurrence of pain after initial improvement suggests premature return to activity or the possibility of litigation.

PHYSICAL EXAMINATION

Physical examination reveals a well-developed, slightly obese female who walks without a limp. Injuries were limited to the neck and right shoulder and did not involve the lower extremities. **She demonstrates limited forward flexion and incomplete extension of the cervical spine. There is decreased motion on right lateral rotation. Cervical range of motion is otherwise full.** One expects some decreased motion after a cervical sprain. **The upper extremities demonstrate normal contours and no atrophy.** A rotator cuff problem of long-standing duration is not present. **There is point tenderness along the right anterior acromial border.** Anterior acromial tenderness and the presence of pain on humeral forward flexion are suggestive of impingement of a swollen rotator cuff on the acromion during abduction and forward flexion. We do not know if the edematous rotator cuff represents aggravation of a preexisting injury or a new injury. **Passive range of motion of the right shoulder is comfortable except on forward flexion beyond 90°, when there is pain in the acromial region.** This is a positive impingement sign, the significance of which is explained above. **Upper extremity motor and sensory tests reveal no deficits.** Neither a cervical neurologic injury nor a significant rotator cuff tear is present. **Supination of the forearm against resistance (Yergason's test for bicipital tendinitis) is painless.** Bicipital tendinitis is not present. Neck pain can refer to the shoulder and vice versa. In this case, the two appear to be unrelated, as there are positive physical findings in both areas suggesting problems in each.

LABORATORY FINDINGS

Radiographs of the cervical spine (not shown) are normal. The normal x-rays rule out an odontoid fracture, cervical vertebral fracture, and facet subluxation. Assessment of ligamentous damage and vertebral instability may require flexion-extension views of the cervical spine. **Fig 9.1 shows AP radiographs of the patient's right shoulder in external (left) and internal (right) rotation views.** A normal right shoulder film eliminates degenerative joint disease of the glenohumeral joint, acromioclavicular joint arthritis or separation, and humeral head/neck fracture.

Shoulder Pain

HISTORY

A 60-year-old right-handed male white-collar worker presents with left shoulder pain of approximately 3 months' duration. The onset was insidious and not related to a particular traumatic incident or period of excessive use. The pain is diffuse, does not radiate, and is particularly bothersome at night, when it has a deep, aching quality. There has been no upper extremity numbness or weakness. A course of anti-inflammatory drugs has not been successful in relieving the pain, which is gradually becoming worse.

PHYSICAL EXAMINATION

Physical examination reveals a healthy-appearing white male holding his left arm against his chest. He removes his shirt with great difficulty. Inspection reveals some atrophy of the spinatus muscles of the left shoulder when compared with the right. There is no point tenderness. Examination of the neck shows full range of motion. Strength testing is inhibited by pain and attempted motion. The right shoulder is normal. Yergason's test for bicipital tendinitis is negative bilaterally. The range of motion and strength of the elbows, wrists, and hands are symmetrical. Active shoulder range of motion examination reveals the following:

	Right	Left
Abduction	180°	50°
Forward flexion	180°	50°
Internal rotation	To T-7	To hip pocket
External rotation	40°	10°

LABORATORY FINDINGS

X-rays of both shoulders (not shown) including AP views in internal and external rotation and an axillary view show normal bony architecture. An AP arthrogram of the left shoulder was taken and is presented in Fig 9.2.

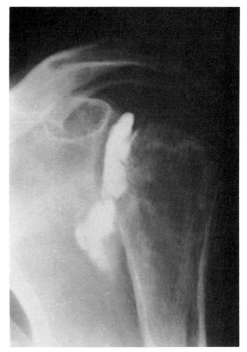

Figure 9.2

QUESTIONS

1. How do you differentiate between arthritis and soft-tissue problems about the shoulder?
2. How can such a condition develop in a white-collar worker who is right-handed and does not subject his left arm to any kind of excessive use?
3. What are the pathomechanics of the stiff, painful shoulder?
4. How could the shoulder stiffness go unnoticed by the patient for 3 months?

Discussion

HISTORY

A 60-year-old right-handed male white-collar worker presents with left shoulder pain of approximately 3 months' duration. The onset was insidious and not related to a particular traumatic incident or period of excessive use. Trauma to the shoulder produces immediate pain following the incident. Excessive use of the shoulder is usually followed by discomfort within 24 hours. Insidious pain is more apt to be associated with degenerative changes or soft-tissue contractures within the shoulder joint or may be referred. **The pain is diffuse, does not radiate, and is particularly bothersome at night, when it has a deep, aching quality.** Structural injury produces localized pain. The lack of radiation suggests that this pain is not originating from the brachial plexus or the cervical spine. Most pain is more apparent at night, but many sources of shoulder pain are aggravated when

the shoulder is slept upon. **There has been no upper extremity numbness or weakness.** A neurologic deficit is unlikely. **A course of anti-inflammatory drugs has not been successful in relieving the pain, which is gradually becoming worse.** The process is not an inflammatory one.

PHYSICAL EXAMINATION

Physical examination reveals a healthy-appearing white male holding his left arm against his chest. He removes his shirt with great difficulty. Range of motion is either painful or restricted or both. **Inspection reveals some atrophy of the spinatus muscles of the left shoulder when compared with the right.** Atrophy of the spinatus muscles can be due to either disuse, rotator cuff tear, or neurologic deficit involving the suprascapular nerve or the C-5 and C-6 roots. **There is no point tenderness.** This rules out acromioclavicular joint arthritis and subacromial bursitis. **Examination of the neck shows full range of motion.** The neck as a source of radiating pain to the shoulder is unlikely. **Strength testing is inhibited by pain and attempted motion.** Strength testing is not reliable. **The right shoulder is normal.** This is a unilateral process. **Yergason's test for bicipital tendinitis is negative bilaterally.** Yergason's test consists of having the patient supinate the forearm against resistance. The biceps tendon is the major supinator of the forearm, and the test will be painful in the presence of bicipital tendinitis. **Range of motion and strength of the elbows, wrists, and hands are symmetrical.** The process is limited to the left shoulder and does not involve the C-5 or C-6 nerve roots. **Active shoulder range of motion examination reveals** 111

the following: (see chart). There is marked restriction of shoulder motion in all planes.

LABORATORY FINDINGS

X-rays of both shoulders (not shown) including AP views in internal and external rotation and an axillary view show normal bony architecture. Degenerative joint disease, loose bodies, and other structural abnormalities are not present. **An AP arthrogram of the left shoulder was taken and is presented in Fig 9.2.** The arthrogram shows diminished capsular space, which can be caused by inadequate filling of the joint space on arthrogram or by a contracted capsule. One of the causes of this is adhesive capsulitis or "frozen shoulder." Adhesive capsulitis may occur insidiously and with no obvious etiology. It may also follow trauma, referred pain to the shoulder (e.g., angina), and immobilization of the shoulder. When the shoulder is immobile for any of these reasons, stiffness and contractures occur. These contractures produce pain when shoulder movement is attempted. Stiffness in the nondominant shoulder often goes unnoticed.

10   Elbow Pain

Elbow Pain

Precipitating Event or Cause	Differential Diagnosis	Key Findings	Key Tests	Natural History if Untreated	Treatment	Expected Outcome with Treatment

Insidious
Increased activity
Occupational overuse
Recreational overuse
Contusion
Previous injury
Neuropathic disorder
  Syringomyelia
  Tabes dorsalis
  Diabetes mellitus
  Leprosy
	DJD	Activity-related pain	X-ray	Progression	NSAID
					- - - - - - - -
					Fusion
						Progression
						- - - - - - - -
						Pain relief

	Bursitis	Red, swollen olecranon bursa	Aspirate Culture Crystal analysis	Acute: resolution, may recur Chronic: recurrence	Splinting Steroids or NSAID if not septic Excision if chronic	Resolution Resolution
	Epicondylitis Tendinitis (tennis elbow)	Tender epicondyle Pain with use of extensors or flexors against resistance		Resolution may recur	NSAID (Ice) Decreased activity	Resolution
	RA	Polyarticular morning stiffness	Positive RF ANA	Variable progression	NSAID Steroids Gold Penicillamine - - - - - - - - Synovectomy	Variable progression Possible joint destruction - - - - - - - - Retard progression
	Osteochondritis dissecans (Little Leaguer's elbow)	Tender condyle	X-ray	Loose bodies DJD	Rest	Resolution

DJD, degenerative joint disease; NSAID, nonsteroidal anti-inflammatory drugs; RA, rheumatoid arthritis; RF, rheumatoid factor; ANA, antinuclear antibodies.

114

Precipitating Event or Cause	Differential Diagnosis	Key Findings	Key Tests	Natural History if Untreated	Treatment	Expected Outcome with Treatment
Insidious Increased activity Occupational overuse Recreational overuse Contusion Previous injury Neuropathic disorder Syringomyelia Tabes dorsalis Diabetes mellitus Leprosy	Loose bodies	Locking	Arthrogram Arthroscopy	Progression	Removal	Improvement
	Referred pain	Neck or shoulder findings	EMG/NCV C-spine x-rays Shoulder x-rays	Recurrence	Treat site of origin of pain	Depends on diagnosis at site of origin of pain
	Neuropathic joint	Swelling Deformity Joint laxity	X-ray	Progressive destruction and instability	Bracing	Progressive joint destruction
	Gout	Exquisite tenderness	Joint fluid crystal analysis Serum uric acid Response to colchicine	Recurrence	NSAID Colchicine Allopurinol Dietary changes	Tendency to recur

NSAID, nonsteroidal anti-inflammatory drugs. EMG, electromyography; NCV, nerve conduction velocity.

HISTORY

A 41-year-old businessman and recreational baritone horn player complains of left elbow pain of 6 weeks' duration. The pain began gradually after the patient joined several brass bands. He is unable to hold his instrument for more than several minutes without severe pain developing about the elbow. The horn is held by the left arm and played with the right hand. The pain is aggravated by elbow extension. Bumping the elbow produces excruciating pain. There has been no trauma. Three weeks ago the patient was treated with anti-inflammatory medication, and his elbow was placed in a posterior splint. The pain has since improved but has not disappeared. General medical history is negative.

PHYSICAL EXAMINATION

Physical examination of both elbows simultaneously reveals no joint effusion or swelling of the olecranon bursae. The left elbow is slightly warmer than the right. Exquisite tenderness is present just proximal to the tip of the olecranon. Extension of the elbow against resistance produces pain.

LABORATORY FINDINGS

Hematocrit is 45, white blood cell count is 8,500, differential is normal, and ESR is 9. X-rays of the elbow (not shown) are normal.

QUESTIONS

1. What findings help you distinguish a local problem from a systemic problem?
2. How do you detect an elbow effusion?
3. Explain the influence of the patient's musical activity on the presenting problem.

Discussion

HISTORY

A 41-year-old businessman and recreational baritone horn player complains of left elbow pain of 6 weeks' duration. The pain began gradually after the patient joined several brass bands. The problem is probably related to playing the baritone horn. **He is unable to hold his instrument for more than several minutes without severe pain developing about the elbow.** The pain is related either to maintaining the elbow in a flexed position, to supporting the weight of the instrument, or to using the wrist and finger muscles, which originate at the elbow. **The horn is held by the left arm and played with the right hand.** This eliminates the wrist and finger muscles as a source of pain. **The pain is aggravated by elbow extension.** The pain could be caused by a loose body within the elbow blocking extension, but we have no evidence of mechanical impingement. This pain could also be originating in the triceps mechanism. **Bumping the elbow produces excruciating pain.** A problem external to the joint would be aggravated by bumping. **There has been no trauma.** This further supports the relationship of the problem to the use of the arm while playing the baritone horn. **Three weeks ago the patient was treated with anti-inflammatory medication, and his elbow was placed in a posterior splint. The pain has since improved but has not disappeared.** An inflammatory component is partly responsible. **General medical history is negative.** A systemic etiology is unlikely.

PHYSICAL EXAMINATION

Physical examination of both elbows simultaneously reveals no joint effusion or swelling of the olecranon bursae. Both olecranon bursitis and intra-articular inflammation have been ruled out. Both elbows should be flexed to 90° in front of the patient and examined at the same time so that the involved side can be compared with the normal side. Effusion of the elbow is best seen and palpated just lateral to the olecranon when the elbow is flexed to 90°. **The left elbow is slightly warmer than the right.** An inflammatory process is present in the more superficial structures. **Exquisite tenderness is present just proximal to the tip of the olecranon.** The triceps surae inserts there. **Extension of the elbow against resistance produces pain.** Use of an inflamed tendon against resistance often produces pain at its insertion.

LABORATORY FINDINGS

Hematocrit is 45, white blood cell count is 8,500, differential is normal, and ESR is 9. X-rays of the elbow (not shown) are normal. A significant septic intra-articular process is not present.

HISTORY

S.C. is a 39-year-old male attorney who complains of right elbow pain that has lasted for approximately 5 months. The problem began after he continued to use a tennis racket that had cracked. The pain was initially felt on the outer side of the elbow and did not radiate. It occurred only during tennis but was not associated with any particular stroke. He has seen another physician, who twice injected cortisone into the painful area. Although the injections decreased the pain somewhat, he was unable to play. Neither acupuncture nor a new racket has improved his condition.

PHYSICAL EXAMINATION

Physical examination reveals a well-muscled individual. There is no evidence of swelling, redness, or deformity of the right elbow. The lateral epicondyle of the elbow is tender to palpation. Passive rotation of the radial head is painless. Wrist dorsiflexion is painful, as is finger extension against resistance. Wrist flexion and finger flexion are painless, and upper extremity sensation is normal.

QUESTIONS

1. In what ways is the elbow prone to injury in athletic activity?
2. What are the pathomechanics of racket-related injury?
3. What nonathletic activities can cause a similar problem?

Discussion

HISTORY

S.C. is a 39-year-old male attorney who complains of right elbow pain that has lasted for approximately 5 months. The problem began after he continued to use a tennis racket that had cracked. A good tennis racket absorbs the impact of the tennis ball. The forces on the patient's arm are determined by the size, construction, stringing, and balance of the racket. These forces will be increased by a defective racket. **The pain was initially felt on the outer side of the elbow and did not radiate.** This suggests that the injury is either musculotendinous or bony in origin and is not likely to be neural. **It occurred only during tennis but was not associated with any particular stroke.** Since all of the muscles that move the wrist and control grip strength and finger motion originate at the elbow, the elbow is particularly susceptible to injury or tendinitis from racket-related sports or any activities that involve wrist motion or gripping. The elbow can also be injured from direct blows during athletic activity. **He has seen another physician, who twice injected cortisone into the painful area.** Cortisone may be useful as a local anti-inflammatory agent. **Although the injections decreased the pain somewhat, he was unable to play. Neither acupuncture nor a new racket has improved his condition.** The lack of response to the above measures indicates that the problem is either noninflammatory (e.g., a stress fracture) or has reached a chronic state.

PHYSICAL EXAMINATION

Physical examination reveals a well-muscled individual. There is no evidence of swelling, redness, or deformity of the right elbow. This eliminates an acute inflammatory process. **The lateral epicondyle of the elbow is tender to palpation.** The origin of the wrist extensor muscles is a common site of tendinitis in racket sports. **Passive rotation of the radial head is painless.** The 'orbicular ligament is not involved. **Wrist dorsiflexion is painful, as is finger extension against resistance.** Tendinitis of the common extensor origin is likely. **Wrist flexion and finger flexion are painless, and upper extremity sensation is normal.** Painless stretch of the extensor origin suggests that no contractures are present. Normal sensation suggests that the problem is not likely to be neural in origin. The same presenting problem can be caused by other activities that involve repetitive wrist and finger movement, such as playing musical instruments, painting, typing, and gardening.

HISTORY

K.G. is a 52-year-old right-handed man complaining of exquisite right elbow pain of 6 hours' duration. In the last few hours the pain has increased markedly in intensity to the point where the patient is unwilling to move his right arm. Twenty-four hours ago the patient underwent carpal tunnel release in his right hand.

The patient's history includes similar episodes of exquisite pain in the wrist and foot. These episodes responded to anti-inflammatory medication. The patient has a history of renal stones.

PHYSICAL EXAMINATION

Physical examination reveals a slightly obese male with a temperature of 99°F. His right elbow is bright red, warm, and swollen posteriorly. It is diffusely tender to palpation. An effusion is present and the patient is unwilling to move his elbow. The surgical dressing on his right wrist is dry, unstained, and nonodorous. There are no erythematous streaks on the arm between the wrist and the elbow. There is no axillary lymphadenopathy. The fingers appear normal.

QUESTIONS

1. How do you distinguish between tendinitis, cellulitis, bursitis, and arthritis?
2. How might the recent surgical procedure be related to the presenting problem?
3. What test or tests are required to make a definitive diagnosis?
4. How might you explain the patient's renal stones?

Discussion

HISTORY

K.G. is a 52-year-old right-handed man complaining of exquisite right elbow pain of 6 hours' duration. The intensity of the pain suggests an acute inflammatory problem. **In the last few hours the pain has increased markedly in intensity to the point where the patient is unwilling to move his right arm.** This acute process is worsening. **Twenty-four hours ago the patient underwent carpal tunnel release in his right hand.** A postoperative streptococcal infection must be considered.

The patient's history includes similar episodes of exquisite pain in the wrist and foot. This suggests that the patient may have a systemic inflammatory problem. **These episodes responded to anti-inflammatory medication.** This confirms the impression above. **The patient has a history of renal stones.** Renal stones can be composed of many different substances including uric acid. Gout should be considered.

PHYSICAL EXAMINATION

Physical examination reveals a slightly obese male with a temperature of 99°F. The temperature suggests that the process is either a low-grade infection or an inflammatory process. Infection in the immediate postoperative period is commonly streptococcal and produces a higher fever. **His right elbow is bright red, warm, and swollen posteriorly.** The redness, warmth, and swelling are consistent with either inflammation or infection. Olecranon bursal swelling is well circumscribed and is located posteriorly over the olecranon, whereas elbow effusions present posterolaterally. **It is diffusely tender to palpation.** The diffuse tenderness suggests that the problem may involve the entire joint rather than the bursa or a superficial tendon. **An effusion is present and the patient is unwilling to move his elbow.** The process involves intra-artic-ular rather than superficial structures. **The surgical dressing on his right wrist is dry, unstained, and nonodorous.** There is no evidence for a grossly purulent infectious process. **There are no erythematous streaks on the arm between the wrist and the elbow. There is no axillary lymphadenopathy.** Cellulitis is not present. **The fingers appear normal.** Wrist infections usually produce finger swelling.

Surgery can be complicated by postoperative infection. It can also precipitate an attack of gout. One must aspirate the joint and examine the fluid for bacteria and uric acid crystals in order to distinguish gout from sepsis.

11

Hand Tingling/ Numbness

Hand Tingling/Numbness

Precipitating Event or Cause	Differential Diagnosis	Key Findings	Key Tests	Natural History if Untreated	Treatment	Expected Outcome with Treatment

Nerve compression or stretch from abnormal posture or position (overhead work, backpacking, leaning on elbow)
Trauma
Occupational overuse
Cervical rib
Insidious (no overt event)
Neuropathy secondary to underlying disease
  leprosy
  tabes dorsalis
  syringomyelia
  RA
  dialysis
  diabetes mellitus
  hypothyroidism
  lead poisoning
  dietary deficiency
  alcoholism
Hysteria
Cigarette smoking
Nerve entrapment or impingement
	Cervical radiculopathy	Neck pain with upper extremity radiation
		Root-specific neurologic sign(s)
			C-spine x-ray
			EMG and NCV
				Intermittent symptoms
				Progression
					Collar and traction
					Fusion
						Improvement

	Thoracic outlet syndrome	Positive Adson's test	X-ray	Intermittent symptoms	Postural training Muscle strengthening Rib removal	Resolution
	Pancoast tumor	History of heavy smoking Supraclavicular fullness Multiple nerve involvement	Apical lordotic x-ray	Progression	Depends on tumor type	Depends on tumor response
	Nerve entrapment at elbow	Tinel's sign at elbow Weakness of muscles above wrist Appropriate sensory deficit	EMG and NCV	Progression	Surgical release or transposition Treat underlying disease	Improvement with early treatment

EMG, electromyography; NCV, nerve conduction velocity; RA, rheumatoid arthritis.

Precipitating Event or Cause	Differential Diagnosis	Key Findings	Key Tests	Natural Course if Untreated	Treatment	Expected Outcome with Treatment

Nerve compression or stretch from abnormal posture or position (overhead work, backpacking, leaning on elbow)
Trauma
Occupational overuse
Cervical rib
Insidious (no overt event)
Neuropathy secondary to underlying disease
  leprosy
  tabes dorsalis
  syringomyelia
  RA
  dialysis
  diabetes mellitus
  hypothyroidism
  lead poisoning
  dietary deficiency
  alcoholism
Hysteria
Cigarette smoking
Nerve entrapment or impingement
	Nerve entrapment at wrist	Tinel's sign in hand
		Increased symptoms with prolonged wrist flexion
		Intrinsic muscle wasting and weakness
		Appropriate sensory deficit
			EMG and NCV	Progression or resolution	Splint
					Surgical release
					Treat underlying disease
						Improvement with early treatment

	Hyperventilation	Uncontrollable tachypnea	Rebreathing in a paper bag	Gradual recovery	Rebreathing	Resolution
	Metabolic neuropathy	Generalized numbness not corresponding to root(s) or peripheral nerve(s)	EMG	Progressive	Treat underlying disease	A function of underlying disease
	Hypothenar hammer syndrome	Positive Allen's test Use of hand as hammer	Arteriogram	Persistent	Arterial ligation	Improvement
	Acute compartmental syndrome	Extreme pain Pain on passive stretch of involved muscles	Compartmental pressure measurement	Ischemic necrosis and contractures	Fasciotomy	Resolution if treated before 12 hours

EMG, electromyography; RA, rheumatoid arthritis.

HISTORY

The patient, a 50-year-old Cambodian, is a right-handed carpenter who comes in complaining of severe right hand and arm pain. Six hours previously he was working on a barn and fell from a ladder, landing on his outstretched right arm. Four hours ago he underwent closed reduction of right midshaft radius and ulna fractures and was sent home with his right arm in a splint and sling. He comes in now because the pain has become steadily worse such that his pain medication is no longer providing any relief.

PHYSICAL EXAMINATION

Physical examination reveals a greatly distressed, robust-appearing male, holding his splinted right arm close to his body. His temperature is 99°F. His arm is wrapped but his thumb and fingers can be examined. They are markedly swollen and cool. The palmar aspects of the patient's thumb and index finger are numb. Sensation in the first dorsal web space and fifth finger is normal. The patient is able to actively flex his fingers within a limited range but refuses to extend them. Passive extension of the fingers produces pain in the forearm. The patient is unable to flex his thumb. The patient is able to abduct and adduct his fingers with equal strength in his right and left hands.

The splint is removed carefully. The forearm is quite swollen and tense, particularly volarly. A small puncture wound, surrounded by dried blood, is present on the volar aspect of the forearm 2 inches proximal to the distal wrist crease. Exquisite tenderness is present on palpation

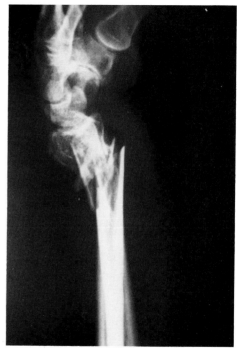

Figure 11.1

of the radius and ulna both volarly and dorsally. The radial pulse is normal.

LABORATORY FINDINGS

A lateral x-ray is shown of the distal right forearm and wrist prior to reduction (Fig 11.1).

QUESTIONS

1. How might you explain the findings noted on sensory and motor examination?
2. What is the significance of:
   A. Pain on passive finger extension?
   B. Normal radial pulse?
   C. Puncture wound?
3. What is the relationship between the site at which the accident occurred, the mechanism of injury, and the current problem?
4. What diagnostic procedures would be useful?

Discussion

HISTORY

The patient, a 50-year-old Cambodian, is a right-handed carpenter who comes in complaining of severe right hand and arm pain. Six hours previously he was working on a barn and fell from a ladder, landing on his outstretched right arm. The energy of injury may be substantial given the height from which the patient fell. Falls on the outstretched arm can produce fractures or dislocations of the carpal bones, radius and ulna, elbow, and shoulder. **Four hours ago he underwent closed reduction of right midshaft radius and ulna fractures and was sent home with his arm in a splint and sling. He comes in now because the pain has become steadily worse such that his pain medication is no longer providing any relief.** Generally, once a fracture is reduced and immobilized, the associated pain should decrease. Increasing pain suggests a complication.

PHYSICAL EXAMINATION

Physical examination reveals a greatly distressed, robust-appearing male, holding his splinted right arm close to his body. His temperature is 99°F. The low-grade temperature suggests a possible inflammatory or infectious process. **His arm is wrapped but his thumb and fingers can be examined. They are markedly swollen and cool.** The swelling and coolness may be due to impaired perfusion from an arterial injury, constrictive dressings, or the position of the limb (90° of elbow flexion). **The palmar aspects of the patient's thumb and index fingers are numb.** The median nerve is impaired. **Sensation in the first dorsal web space and fifth finger is normal.** Radial and ulnar nerve sensory function remains normal. **The patient is able to actively flex his fingers within a limited range but refuses to extend them. Passive extension of the fingers produces pain in the forearm.** Partial active finger flexion makes direct median nerve injury or tendon injury less likely than impairment due to ischemia. Pain with passive extension is consistent with a developing acute anterior compartmental syndrome. Ischemic muscles are painful when stretched. **The patient is unable to flex his thumb.** The anterior interosseous nerve innervates the flexor pollicis longus in the anterior compartment. The flexor pollicis longus also could have been injured by the fracture fragments. **The patient is able to abduct and adduct his**

127

fingers with equal strength in his right and left hands. The ulnar nerve is intact.

The splint is removed carefully. The forearm is quite swollen and tense, particularly volarly. Moderate swelling is normal after a fracture. Tense swelling, especially volarly, is consistent with an acute compartmental syndrome. A small puncture wound, surrounded by dried blood, is present on the volar aspect of the forearm 2 inches proximal to the distal wrist crease. This fracture is technically "open" (compound). The fractured bones probably punctured the skin from within. Knowing that the patient fell near a barn, we must consider potential contamination of the fracture with Gram-negative or anaerobic organisms. Because the patient is Cambodian, he may not have had tetanus prophylaxis. Although the high energy of injury associated with a fall from a height can produce an acute compartmental syndrome, the possibil-

ity of swelling from arterial injury or gas-producing organisms must be considered. Exquisite tenderness is present on palpation of the radius and ulna both volarly and dorsally. The site of an acute fracture is normally tender. The radial pulse is normal. Normal pulses do not rule out arterial injury or compartmental syndromes.

LABORATORY FINDINGS

A lateral x-ray of the distal right forearm and wrist was obtained (Fig 11.1). The lateral x-ray reveals angulated fractures of the distal radius and ulna with the apex facing volarly. Compartmental pressure measurements, arteriograms, and Gram stain of the wound would all provide useful additional information. However, given the rapidly progressing deficits, the patient should be taken to the operating room and the arm opened, decompressed, and débrided.

Hand Tingling/Numbness

Case 30. 30-Year-Old Pregnant Typist

HISTORY

The patient is a 30-year-old female typist with a 3-month history of aching and progressive numbness in the entire left hand. The numbness is worse at night. The right hand also becomes numb at night, but the numbness is relieved by shaking the hand over the side of the bed. The patient has been treated with wrist splints, which have not improved the symptoms. She is pregnant and expecting her baby in 1 month.

PHYSICAL EXAMINATION

No thenar, hypothenar, or intrinsic muscle wasting is evident. Sensation of light touch is normal. The smallest distance at which the patient can distinguish two simultaneously applied pinpoints (two-point discrimination) is 3 mm on all the fingertips of the right hand and 5 mm on the left. Strength in both hands is normal. Tapping over the carpal tunnel does not produce paresthesias in a median nerve distribution (negative Tinel's sign). Forced volar flexion of the wrist (Phalen's test) produces bilateral hand pain and numbness in the median nerve distribution.

LABORATORY FINDINGS

Electrodiagnostic studies reveal the following results:

	Left	Right
Median nerve motor latency across the wrist	4.8 sec	4.9 sec
Median nerve sensory latency across the wrist	5.3 sec	4.6 sec
Ulnar sensory latencies across the wrist	3.4 sec	3.1 sec
Nerve conduction velocity from the elbow to the wrist	52 meters/sec	52 meters/sec
Insertional activity in the abductor pollicis brevis	Increased	Increased

QUESTIONS

1. How do you distinguish a local problem at the wrist from a more proximal one?
2. Why is the problem worse at night?
3. What effect is the pregnancy having on this patient's problem?

Discussion

HISTORY

The patient is a 30-year-old female typist wih a 3-month history of aching and progressive numbness in the entire left hand. Forward posture of the neck may cause cervical nerve impingement and referred pain. Extremes of wrist volar or dorsiflexion may cause impingement of the median nerve in the carpal tunnel. Numbness in the entire hand is unusual and may reflect a systemic neuropathy. **The numbness is worse at night. The right hand also becomes numb at night, but the numbness is relieved by shaking the hand over the side of the bed.** This is very characteristic of a carpal tunnel syndrome. Hyperflexion of the wrist, which can occur in sleep, compresses the median nerve. Numbness from neuropathy is persistent and not affected by time of day or wrist position. **The patient has been treated with wrist splints, which have not improved the symptoms.** Wrist position is not causing the problem. **She is pregnant and expecting her baby in 1 month.** Hypervolemia of pregnancy can cause swelling in the carpal tunnel and therefore may be responsible for the symptoms.

PHYSICAL EXAMINATION

No thenar, hypothenar, or intrinsic muscle wasting is evident. Sensation of light touch is normal. Nerve involvement is not severe or long-standing. **The smallest distance at which the patient can distinguish two simultaneously applied pinpoints (two-point discrimination) is 3 mm on all the fingertips of the right hand and 5 mm on the left.** The two-point discrimination test is the most sensitive test for early sensory loss. The distance at which two points can be distinguished is usually 2 to 3 mm or less on the fingertips and becomes larger as one proceeds toward the palm. This patient's two-point discrimination is abnormal only in her left hand. **Strength in both hands is normal.** This is further evidence that the problem is not severe. **Tapping over the carpal tunnel does not produce paresthesias in a median nerve distribution (negative Tinel's sign).** Percussing an irritated nerve will produce paresthesias in the distribution of that nerve. **Forced volar flexion of the wrist (Phalen's test)** **produces bilateral hand pain and numbness in the median nerve distribution.** This test reproduces the hyperflexion that is probably occurring at night and compressing the median nerve in the carpal tunnel. Hyperflexion may cause symptoms but not be the etiology of the problem.

LABORATORY FINDINGS

Electrodiagnostic studies reveal the following: (see chart). This patient's right median sensory latency and bilateral conduction velocities are normal. The left median sensory latency is prolonged. Median motor latencies at the wrist are slightly prolonged bilaterally. Increased insertional activity in the median-innervated muscles suggests irritability and median nerve neuropathy. The normal nerve conduction velocity eliminates systemic neuropathy. The abnormal motor latency at the wrist and the positive Phalen's test suggest a problem originating at the wrist rather than from the neck or the elbow. Decreased sensation in the median nerve distribution, Tinel's sign, Phalen's test, and decreased power in median-innervated muscles are signs of carpal tunnel syndrome. All signs need not be present to make the diagnosis. In this patient, the symptoms, the positive Phalen's test, and the electrodiagnostic findings support the diagnosis of carpal tunnel syndrome.

HISTORY

A 58-year-old right-handed male drifter complains of inability to straighten his left ring and little fingers and his right little finger. He also complains of numbness and tingling in the same digits. These symptoms have been progressive over the last 3 years. At present his left hand bothers him more than his right. Medical history is positive for heavy alcohol intake. He smokes two packs of cigarettes per day.

PHYSICAL EXAMINATION

Physical examination reveals a disheveled, poorly nourished male. Movement of the neck is normal and produces no symptoms. No supraclavicular fullness is noted. Pitting of the palmar fascia is present on the left hand, as is a 60° flexion contracture of the left ring finger metacarpophalangeal joint. The patient has a single pretendinous band along the fourth ray in the palm. The right hand has more severe contractures of the fifth ray, with a 90° contracture of the MCP joint and a volarly subluxed proximal interphalangeal joint. The wrist range of motion is not restricted, and tests for vascular circulation of the hand reveal normal results. The patient has a positive Tinel's sign at the left elbow with paresthesias felt in the hypothenar eminence on the left hand. Hand grip strength is normal bilaterally.

The smallest distance at which the patient can distinguish two simultaneously applied pinpoints (two-point discrimination) is 10 mm on the fourth and fifth fingertips and 5 mm on the tips of the thumb and index fingers of the left hand. The patient is able to sense light touch throughout the left hand. Sensory examination of the right hand reveals a two-point discrimination of 8 mm in the fourth and fifth fingertips and 6 mm in the thumb and index fingertips. Motor strength is normal.

LABORATORY FINDINGS

Electrodiagnostic studies reveal the following:

	Left	Right
Median nerve sensory latency across wrist	4.7 sec	4.6 sec
Median nerve motor latency across wrist	3.8 sec	4.7 sec
Ulnar nerve sensory latency across wrist	11 sec	3.6 sec
Ulnar nerve motor latency across wrist	5.5 sec	3.2 sec
Median nerve conduction velocity across elbow	53 meters/sec	53 meters/sec
Ulnar nerve conduction velocity across elbow	45 meters/sec	50 meters/sec

Apical lordotic chest x-ray (not shown) is normal.

QUESTIONS

1. In a patient who cannot extend his fingers, how do you distinguish between muscle weakness, tenodesis, joint contracture, and palmar fascia contracture?
2. Explain the role of two-point discrimination in the sensory evaluation.
3. How do you differentiate neuropathy from nerve entrapment?

Discussion

HISTORY

A 58-year-old right-handed male drifter complains of inability to straighten his left ring and little fingers and his right little finger. Inability to straighten the fingers can be due to a contracture or lack of extensor motor function. **He also complains of numbness and tingling in the same digits.** These digits are innervated by C-8 via the ulnar nerve. **These symptoms have been progressive over the last 3 years.** A traumatic origin is unlikely. **At present his left hand bothers him more than his right. Medical history is positive for heavy alcohol intake.** Alcoholism is associated with both palmar fascia contracture (Dupuytren's contracture) as well as peripheral neuropathy. **He smokes two packs of cigarettes per day.** Heavy smoking is associated with lung tumors. When these occur in the apex of the lung they can produce medial cord neuropathy in the brachial plexus. The ulnar nerve is a branch of the medial cord.

PHYSICAL EXAMINATION

Physical examination reveals a disheveled, poorly nourished male. Movement of the neck is normal and produces no symptoms. Cervical radiculopathy is unlikely. **No supraclavicular fullness is noted.** Supraclavicular fullness is associated with apical lung tumors and lymphadenopathy. **Pitting of the palmar fascia is present on the left hand, as is a 60° flexion contracture of the left**

ring finger metacarpophalangeal joint. **The patient has a single pretendinous band along the fourth ray in the palm. The right hand has more severe contractures of the fifth ray with a 90° contracture of the MCP joint and a volarly subluxed proximal interphalangeal joint.** These findings are all consistent with contracture of the palmar fascia, which when severe may produce subluxation of the interphalangeal joints. The inability of the patient to straighten his fingers is due to the contractures. Attempts to flex the MCP joints should relax the palmar fascia and lessen the apparent interphalangeal contractures if they are secondary. If the interphalangeal joint itself is contracted, its apparent contracture will not change with MCP joint flexion. **The wrist's range of motion is not restricted, and tests for vascular circulation of the hand reveal normal results.** Normal wrist range of motion rules out a flexor tendon tenodesis as the etiology of the finger flexion contractures. The numbness and tingling are more likely to be neural than vascular in origin. **The patient has a positive Tinel's sign at the left elbow, with paresthesias felt in the hypothenar eminence on the left hand.** Percussing an inflamed nerve produces paresthesias or dysesthesias in the distribution of that nerve. The sign is useful in localizing the site of entrapment, inflammation, nerve regeneration, or neuroma. A positive Tinel's sign in this patient localizes an area of entrapment at the elbow but does not rule out metabolic neuropathy. Compression neuropathies are more common in nerves that are also metabolically compromised. **Hand grip strength is normal bilaterally.** Neuromuscular function is normal.

The smallest distance at which the patient can distinguish two simultaneously applied pinpoints (two-point discrimination) is 10 mm on the fourth and fifth fingertips and 5 mm on the tips of the thumb and index fingers of the left hand. The patient is able to sense light touch throughout the left hand. Two-point discrimination is slightly abnormal in the thumb and index fingers and distinctly abnormal in the fourth and fifth fingers. The two-point discrimination test measures sensory deficit. Sensory examination of the right hand reveals a two-point discrimination of 8 mm in the fourth and fifth fingertips and 6 mm in the thumb and index fingertips. The sensory deficit in the right hand does not seem to be as severe as in the left hand. Motor strength is normal.

LABORATORY FINDINGS

Electrodiagnostic studies reveal the following (see chart). The electrodiagnostic studies of median nerve latency across the wrist reveal normal findings. The ulnar nerve sensory and motor latencies across the wrist are normal in the right hand but significantly prolonged in the left hand. The median nerve conduction velocity across the elbow is normal. The ulnar nerve conduction velocity across the elbow is slowed on the left side. The ulnar nerve is entrapped or injured at both the left elbow and the wrist. When metabolic neuropathy is present, nerve conduction velocity prolongation is not isolated to a specific nerve. Apical lordotic chest x-ray (not shown) is normal. An apical lung tumor is not present.

HISTORY

M.P. is a 31-year-old female masters swimmer who complains of 7 days of discomfort in her neck and numbness radiating into the right index, long, and ring fingers. She denies any weakness. She also has a long history of intermittent mottling and coldness of the right arm. The patient swims predominantly breast stroke as well as a bit of freestyle. Recently she began a training regimen doing a one-armed butterfly stroke with the right arm only.

PHYSICAL EXAMINATION

On physical examination the patient has full forward flexion and extension of her neck. On side bending to the right, the ear fails to reach the shoulder by 1 inch; to the left the ear fails to reach the shoulder by 2 inches, and this movement produces some discomfort in the right trapezius area. Attempting to touch chin to shoulder fails by 1 cm on the right and by 2 cm on the left. No supraclavicular fullness or shoulder girdle atrophy is noted. Range of motion of the shoulder is normal. Sensory and motor examination of her upper extremities is entirely normal. She has a positive Adson's test on the right. Tinel's tests at the elbow and wrist are negative.

LABORATORY FINDINGS

AP (left) and lateral (right) x-ray views of the cervical spine are shown (Fig 11.2).

QUESTIONS

1. What relationship does the patient's swimming have to her current problem?
2. What can cause intermittent mottling and coldness in the upper extremities?
3. What are the most common sites of upper extremity nerve entrapment? What is the approach for determining the site of involvement?

Discussion

HISTORY

M.P. is a 31-year-old female masters swimmer who complains of 7 days of discomfort in her neck and numbness radiating into the right index, long, and ring fingers. The nerve roots innervating the index, long, and ring fingers are C-6 and C-7. The associated neck discomfort suggests that a nerve entrapment may be originating in the cervical spine. **She denies any weakness.** This is a measure of severity of the neural problem. **She also has a long history of intermittent mottling and coldness of the right arm.** These findings can be due to a sympathetic overactivity or to vascular entrapment in the subclavian or thoracic outlet area. In addition, women are often subject to systemic vasculitis. The fact that the mottling and coldness are limited to one arm makes sympathetic overactivity and vasculitis less likely. **The patient swims**

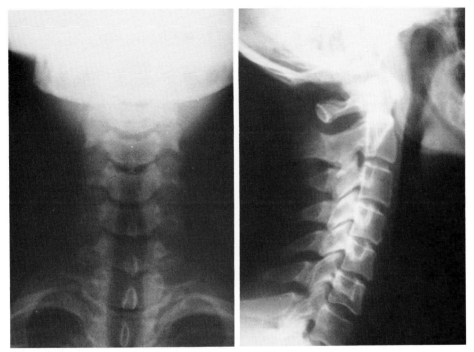

Figure 11.2

predominantly breast stroke as well as a bit of freestyle. **Recently she began a training regimen doing a one-armed butterfly stroke with the right arm only.** Both the butterfly and the breast stroke use the pectoral muscles a great deal. Hypertrophy of the musculature in this area can produce entrapment of the nerves and/or the blood vessels in the thoracic outlet region.

PHYSICAL EXAMINATION

On physical examination the patient has full forward flexion and extension of her neck. On side bending to the right, the ear fails to reach the shoulder by 1 inch; to the left the ear fails to reach the shoulder by 2 inches, and this movement produces some discomfort in the right trapezius area. Attempting to touch chin to shoulder fails by 1 cm on the right and by 2 cm on the left. Restricted range of motion can be due to muscle spasm or degenerative changes in the cervical spine. **No supraclavicular fullness or shoulder girdle atrophy is noted.** Supraclavicular fullness is associated with lymphadenopathy and apical lung tumors, which could also impinge on the neurovascular structures in this area. Shoulder girdle atrophy might be seen with disuse, rotator cuff tear, or suprascapular or cervical nerve root entrapment. **Range of motion of the shoulder is normal.** One cause of neck pain is referred pain from a shoulder problem. The

patient's normal shoulder examination makes this unlikely. **Sensory and motor examination of her upper extremities is entirely normal.** Her nerve involvement is not severe. **She has a positive Adson's test on the right.** When the arm is abducted and the head rotated, any abnormal constriction of the vascular structures in the thoracic outlet will be increased. **Tinel's tests at the elbow and wrist are negative.** Percussing a nerve is unlikely to produce tingling (Tinel's sign) in the case of generalized neuropathy but is helpful in determining the site of involvement of nerve entrapment or impingement. In the upper extremity, the most common sites of nerve entrapment include the cervical spine, the thoracic outlet, the elbow, and the wrist. The median, ulnar, and radial nerves can also become entrapped in the forearm musculature, although this is less common. The site of nerve entrapment can be determined by physical findings and electrodiagnostic tests.

LABORATORY FINDINGS

AP (left) and lateral (right) x-ray views of the cervical spine are shown (Fig 11.2). These x-rays reveal no abnormalities. Thoracic outlet syndrome is often associated with an accessory cervical rib or a fibrous band extending from a rudimentary cervical rib. Both of these anomalous structures can produce traction on the brachial plexus.

GLOSSARY

GLOSSARY

Abductor lurch

An abnormal gait seen in the presence of hip abductor muscle weakness. When the patient's weight is on the involved leg during stance phase, the trunk will lurch toward the involved side.

Adson's test

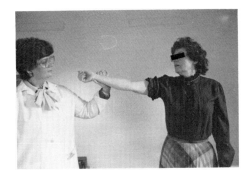

A test for impingement of vascular structures at the thoracic outlet. The patient's arm is gradually elevated in an abduction arc while the examiner's fingers are held on the patient's radial pulse. As the arm is abducted, the patient is asked to turn the head away from the tested side and take a deep breath. If the pulse disappears as the arm is abducted beyond 90°, the test is positive for impingement. The test can be repeated with the head turned toward the side being examined.

Alkaline phosphatase

A laboratory measurement of bone turnover.

Allen's test

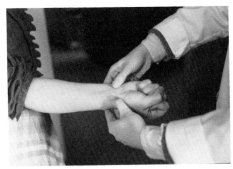

A test for integrity of the radial and ulnar arteries at the wrist. The examiner compresses the patient's radial and ulnar arteries at the wrist. The patient is then asked to open and close the hand rapidly until the palm appears white. The examiner then releases either the radial or the ulnar artery and looks for return of pink color and circulation to the hand. The test is then repeated releasing the other artery. The hand should return to its pink color within 6 seconds if circulation through that artery is adequate.

ANA

Antinuclear antibody. A laboratory test for autoimmune disease.

Ankle mortise

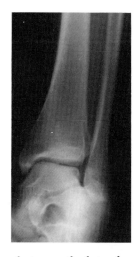

The space between the lateral and medial malleoli into which the talus projects.

139

Arthrogram

A radiologic study in which radiopaque contrast material is injected into a joint. Useful in delineating soft-tissue pathology within the joint.

Arthroscopy

A technique in which a fiberoptic periscope-like structure (arthroscope) is inserted into a joint for direct visualization of the interior of the joint.

Arthrotomograms

Tomograms taken during arthrography. Tomography is a special technique that shows in detail the images of structures lying in a predetermined plane of tissue while blurring detail of structures in other planes.

AVN

Avascular necrosis. Death of tissue due to lack of blood supply.

Bamboo spine

The appearance on x-ray of the spine of a person who has had ankylosing spondylitis for many years. The calcification that has occurred between vertebral bodies at the edges of the disk gives the appearance of a bamboo stalk. Anteroposterior (top) and lateral (bottom) views of the lumbar spine illustrate the phenomenon.

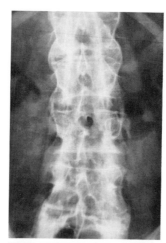

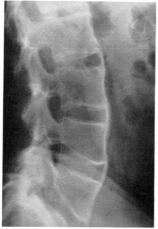

Bamboo spine

Cavus foot

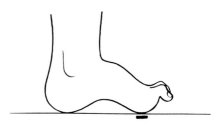

A foot that is rather inflexible and has an abnormally high arch.

CBC

Complete blood count. Usually includes white blood cell count, hematocrit, hemoglobin, platelet count, and indices of red blood cell size and hemoglobin concentration.

Chest expansion test

A test that measures the difference in chest circumference between maximal inspiration and maximal expiration. The difference usually exceeds 2 inches.

Claw toes

Toes in which the metatarsophalangeal joint is hyperextended and the proximal and distal interphalangeal joints are flexed.

Core decompression

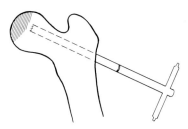

A procedure to prevent collapse of the avascular area in patients with avascular necrosis of the femoral head. Removing a core of bone from the femoral head and neck decreases the elevated interosseous pressure.

CT scan

Computed tomography scan. A computerized method of reconstituting tomographic x-rays of a structure such that it can be examined in frontal or sagittal planes or in cross section.

de Quervain's disease

Tenosynovitis of the extensor pollicis brevis and abductor pollicis longus tendons.

DJD

Degenerative joint disease. Osteoarthrosis. Osteoarthritis.

Dysrhythmia

Defective rhythm. Motion of the spine that is not smooth in nature but is marked by sudden stops, starts, and/or shifts in direction.

EMG

Electromyography. The recording of changes in the electrical potential of muscle. Useful in determining muscle disease or denervation.

ESR

Erythrocyte sedimentation rate ("sed rate"). The distance (in millimeters) that a defined aliquot of red blood cells settles in 1 hour. A nonspecific test for systemic inflammation.

Eversion

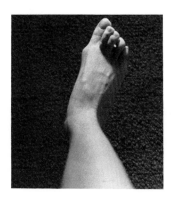

Turning outward. Often used in describing movement of the foot on the ankle. The foot moves away from the midline when it is everted.

Freiberg's infraction

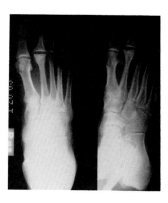

Necrosis of the head of the second metatarsal.

GC

Gonococcus. Used as an abbreviation for gonorrhea, an infection caused by the gonococcal bacteria.

Hallux valgus

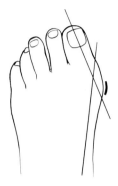

A foot deformity in which the great toe drifts laterally (away from the midline of the body. This angulation is often associated with varus (toward the midline) angulation of the first metatarsal and with bunion formation at the first metatarsal joint.

Hammer toe

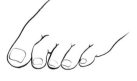

Flexion contracture of the proximal interphalangeal joint, which causes the toe to tap the ground like a hammer.

HLA-B-27

HLA (human lymphocyte antigen) analysis is a method of tissue typing for specific genotypes. The B-27 antigen is a specific antigen associated with spondyloarthropathies.

Hypothenar hammer syndrome

Impairment of ulnar arterial flow to the hand caused by using the base of the palm like a hammer.

Impingement syndrome

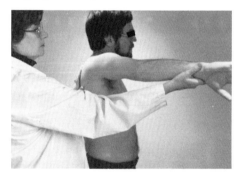

Described by Charles Neer, a syndrome in which pain is produced in the anterior shoulder when the arm is flexed past 90°. Impingement occurs against the anterior edge of the acromion, the coracoacromial ligament, and/or the acromioclavicular joint. A positive impingement test may be associated with subacromial bursitis, acromioclavicular degenerative joint disease, biceps tendinitis, and rotator cuff tears.

Impulse pain

Pain produced by forcefully percussing the distal end of an extremity to produce an impulse wave extending up the extremity. This test is commonly used in the lower extremity and is positive in the presence of fracture somewhere in the lower extremity.

Inversion

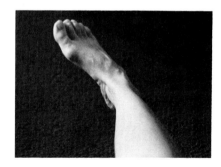

Turning inward. Commonly used to describe motion of the foot on the ankle. The foot moves toward the midline.

Latency

The time (in milliseconds) it takes for an electrical impulse to travel from the point of application to a reference point. Used in association with nerve conduction velocity testing.

List

A nautical term implying leaning of a ship. Used medically to describe leaning of the torso due to involuntary back spasm.

MMPI

Minnesota Multiphasic Personality Inventory. A psychological test useful in patients with chronic pain problems.

Morton's foot

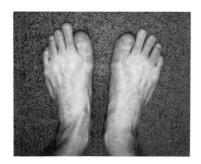

A foot in which the first metatarsal is shorter and more mobile than the second metatarsal.

Morton's neuroma

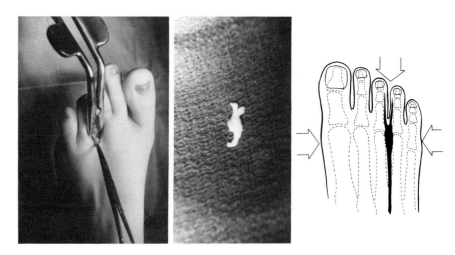

Thickening of the interdigital nerve between the third and fourth interspaces in the foot.

MRI

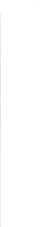

Magnetic resonance imaging. An imaging technique that involves magnetizing and then demagnetizing an anatomical structure. The resonance produced is interpreted by a computer, which generates a multiplanar image of the structure. This technique can demonstrate lesions in cartilage and soft tissue normally invisible on conventional x-ray, and it involves no radiation.

Myelogram

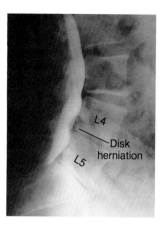

An x-ray of the spine taken following injection of radiopaque dye into the dural sac surrounding the spinal cord. The dye makes the cord and nerve roots visible on the x-ray and may reveal such conditions as tumor, disk herniation, and spinal stenosis.

Nerve conduction velocity

A test that measures the speed or velocity with which a nerve conducts an electrical impulse from the point of application to a reference point. Measured in meters per second.

Pancoast tumor

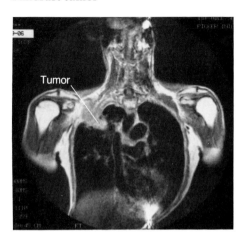

A tumor located in the apex of the lung.

Patrick's sign

A sign of sacroiliac irritation. The sign is elicited in the supine patient by abducting the hip and flexing the knee of one extremity such that the lateral malleolus is placed over the opposite knee. Pressure is then simultaneously applied to the flexed knee and the opposite anterior superior iliac spine. If the test is positive, pain is produced in the sacroiliac joint.

Patrick's sign

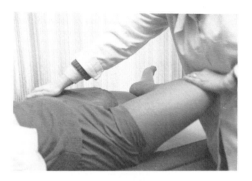

Phalen's test

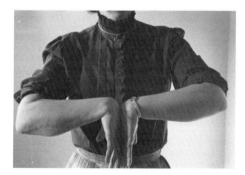

A test for carpal tunnel syndrome in which both hands are held tightly palmar-flexed opposite to a prayer position, creating at least a 90° angle between the forearm and the hand. If the test is positive, numbness and tingling are produced when the hands are held in this position for approximately 30 seconds.

RA
Rheumatoid arthritis. A chronic, systemic inflammatory disorder of unknown etiology characterized by polyarticular, symmetrical joint involvement.

Reiter's syndrome
A triad of arthritis, urethritis, and iritis or conjunctivitis.

Rheumatoid factor
An immunoglobulin antigen-antibody complex often found circulating in the serum of adult patients with rheumatoid arthritis.

Sequestration
The isolation of an area of dead bone from normal bone during the process of septic necrosis.

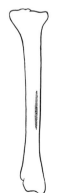

Spondyloarthropathy
An abnormality of the joints in the spine.

Spondylolisthesis

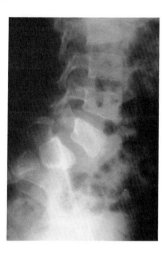

Slipping of a vertebral body, usually in an anterior direction, associated with defects or fractures of the pars interarticularis of the vertebral arch.

Straight leg raising sign

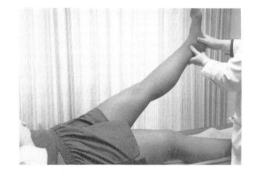

Pain traveling down the ipsilateral leg when the knee is held straight and the entire lower extremity is flexed at the hip.

Cross straight leg raising sign

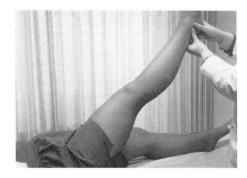

Pain traveling down the opposite leg when the straight leg raising test is performed.

Reverse straight leg raising sign

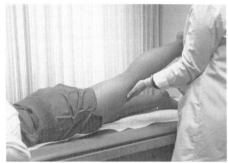

Pain traveling down the ipsilateral leg when the patient is prone and the leg is extended at the hip and the knee.

Tarsal coalition

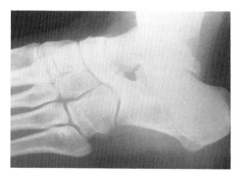

A joining together of two tarsal bones. The coalition can be fibrous, cartilaginous, or bony.

Tenodesis
Fixation of a tendon to bone.

Tension signs
Signs that indicate tension on a nerve root, such as the straight leg raising sign.

Thomas test

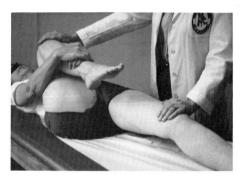

A test for hip flexion contracture. The uninvolved flexed leg is held against the chest of the supine patient to flatten the lumbar lordosis. If a hip flexion contracture is present in the opposite leg it will not remain flush with the examination table. The angle formed between the involved leg and the examination table equals the number of degrees of flexion contracture present.

Transtrochanteric osteotomy

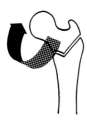

Surgical cutting of the femur through the lesser trochanter. Used to treat avascular necrosis of the femoral head by moving the weight-bearing forces from the necrotic area to a healthy area of the femoral head.

Trendelenburg's sign

A sign of gluteus medius weakness or relative inhibition. The sign is elicited by asking the patient to stand on the involved leg and raise the uninvolved leg. If the sign is positive, the pelvis will drop on the uninvolved side.

WBC count

White blood cell count. A laboratory measurement of the number of leukocytes in 1 mm^3 of blood.

Yergason's test

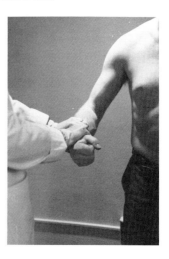

A test for biceps tendinitis in which supination of the forearm is resisted. The test is positive if this resistance produces pain in the biceps tendon.

WORKING DIAGNOSIS KEY

Case 1. Degenerative joint disease
Case 2. Avascular necrosis of the femoral head
Case 3. Femoral neck fracture
Case 4. Gonorrheal arthritis
Case 5. Rheumatoid arthritis
Case 6. Tibial fracture
Case 7. Periosteal sarcoma
Case 8. Osteomyelitis
Case 9. Periostitis of the left tibia and stress fracture of the right tibia
Case 10. Chronic ankle instability
Case 11. Flexor hallucis longus tenosynovitis
Case 12. Osteochondral fracture of the talus
Case 13. Posttraumatic osteoarthritis
Case 14. Metatarsal stress fracture
Case 15. Reiter's syndrome
Case 16. Metatarsalgia
Case 17. Hallux rigidus

Case 18. Morton's neuroma
Case 19. Disc herniation
Case 20. Pain problem
Case 21. Metastatic cancer
Case 22. Spondylolysis
Case 23. Rotator cuff tear
Case 24. Cervical strain and impingement syndrome
Case 25. Adhesive capsulitis
Case 26. Triceps tendinitis
Case 27. Lateral epicondylitis
Case 28. Gout
Case 29. Acute volar compartmental syndrome secondary to gas gangrene
Case 30. Carpal tunnel syndrome
Case 31. Cubital tunnel syndrome and Dupuytren's contracture
Case 32. Thoracic outlet syndrome

INDEX